COFFEE IN THE CEREAL

The First Year with Multiple Sclerosis

BY

Lorna Moorhead

Pathfinder Publishing of California
Oxnard, California

COFFEE IN THE CEREAL

Published By:
Pathfinder Publishing of California
3600 Harbor Boulevard, #82
Oxnard, CA 93035

Libraary of Congress Cataloging-in-Publication Data
Moorhead, Lorna J.
  Coffee In The Cereal
  p.cm
  Includes bibliographical references
ISBN 0-934793-07-7 $14.95

ISBN 0-934-793-07-7

Introduction

In August of 1998 at the age of 23 and in top aerobic shape, I suddenly found myself battling with horrible fatigue. Where I had once been jogging up and down a steep hill to my mailbox, I now didn't have the energy or will to get out of bed. Near the end of the month the tremor in my hands had become much worse and I was beginning to drop things. A year later after being subjected to various hypotheses ranging from hypoglycemic to crazy, I was given a final diagnosis of Multiple Sclerosis.

When I decided to sit down and write *Coffee in The Cereal*, but was floundering for what area to focus on, a dear friend of mine said, "Describe your book in one sentence." In my usual sarcastic fashion I replied: "It's the let me tell you about how I learned to live with MS without making you want to slit your wrists book." So while the diagnostic period was difficult and is chock full of stories, it will have to wait for another book. I wanted *this* book to focus on how **life goes on** once you crawl out from under the sheets and decide to **kick some autoimmune butt**. (And you have my permission to crawl under your sheets because I did it too. I even went on a nice little drinking binge until I "straightened up and flew right." Well I flew more or less in a wavy pattern because most people with MS can't fly straight.)

Coffee in the Cereal is a book for anyone who would like a better idea of what life is like for us average MSers, after the "big dx" of Multiple Sclerosis. (Without all the medical jargon and psychobabble. Not that psychobabble is bad, I just do enough babbling on my own for one book.)

COFFEE IN THE CEREAL – FOREWORD

By Judith Lynn Nichols, author _Women Living With Multiple Sclerosis_ & _Living Beyond Multiple Sclerosis, A Woman's Guide._

Lorna Moorhead grew up with the idea that she doesn't always have to conform to society's norms or expectations. She lives by the conviction that there is always a different way of perceiving things, and just because you don't see something in the same was as everybody else, doesn't mean you're wrong. _Coffee In the Cereal_ is evidence that she practices what she believes.

From the first chapter, when the author equates death, using a wheelchair, or losing the power of speech with ("God forbid!") forgetting her PIN, it's obvious that this book doesn't conform to normal expectations of a report about a chronic, disabling illness.

Lorna doesn't hand us a scholarly treatise on causes and cures, symptoms and treatments of multiple sclerosis. She simply invites us to accompany her on a road filled with "sharp turns, potholes, and near misses," as she makes her way through the first couple of years after her Big Bang first appearance of symptoms and her subsequent diagnosis of MS.

We watch her research the disease, ponder the "holes" in her head, and adopt a morning ritual of checking her pillow to see if her brains leaked out during the night. We hear her react to the reactions to her diagnosis of those around her: the Sergeants, Skeptics, Morticians, Movie Stars, and Mutts (who combine the reactions of all the others).

Explaining multiple sclerosis to her young son (when he noticed that not all mothers move around on their butts) might have been a heartbreaking task.

But we have to laugh as she employs a hot dog in a bun to illustrate a nerve encased in myelin, and invites her son to nibble on it, "not enough to break the hot dog, but to make it rather floppy."

We go with her to a doctor's appointment, where she feels that her complaints are ignored or dismissed and she's nothing but a hypochondriac. ("Hypochondriacs, like Chicken Little, can be very annoying. Sure, the sky might really be falling, but people hate the constant squawking.")

She even invites us into her bedroom, where she's planned a romance-renewing evening with her husband. Her store of enticements includes a fishnet bodysuit that her husband is sure to find irresistible. But MS's coordination problems result in body parts being inserted into inappropriate bodysuit openings, and in Lorna looking like "a netted crab." Once again, we laugh with her at what might otherwise have been a sad situation.

In addition to having the ability to find humor in the humorless aspects of life with MS, Lorna is able to come to peace with and even develop respect for the institutions and individuals who made her adjustment to MS so difficult. Of the medical professionals who seemed unsympathetic to her complaints, she says finally, " A doctor ... does not have the ability to jump into my skin and know how I'm truly feeling. They can't see through my eyes; it was unfair of me to expect them to."

By the end of those first couple of years with MS, Lorna realized that there are many others like her, especially young mothers with MS, who could use a fresh perspective on life with chronic illness. She began, and continues now, to offer support and solidarity *via* MS MOMS, her local and website- based support group where families learn together to manage multiple sclerosis.

Multiple sclerosis is a serious disease, with devastating effects for those who live with it. Lorna Moorhead's writing doesn't try to diminish the gravity of a diagnosis of MS or to minimize the

Forward

devastation MS causes. *Coffee In the Cereal* tries, instead, to get beyond the gravity and the devastation, and offer us a less somber outlook on life with MS.

Early in the book, Lorna tells us, "I resolved to laugh at my MS, to thumb my nose at it, and to live my life exactly as I had before." I hope to read, years from now, that she is able to carry on with that attitude and to continue to share it with others with MS.

Judith Lynn Nichols

Acknowledgments

I would like to thank all those family and friends who had faith in my abilities when creating this book.

In particular:

To Reva Basch, who helped run me through my first drafts and put up with my neuroses.

To John Bryans and Mark Suchomel who both thought my idea worthy enough to pass on

To Bill Mosbrook who decided to give me a shot

To Judith Lynn Nichols who believed it was good enough.

To Mom and Gordon who gave me feedback.

To Dad who didn't think I needed any.

To my husband, Mark, who helped me stay disciplined, put up with my rants when we disagreed on verb-subject agreement, and never quit reminding me how much faith he had in me.

To my MS MOMS who stood behind me even when I faltered (You are so many I can't list you all and I'm so daft I can't remember all your names. *grin *)

And to my son Stephan who still thinks that all I'm doing when I'm at the computer is "playing". I love you.

~LJM

This book is dedicated to all of my MS MOMS

Thank you for understanding and ecourgaing me.

~The Woman Behind the Curtain

Contents

Chapter One

I need you like a hole in the head.

You find out you have MS when your neurologist mistakenly asks, "So what are you taking for your MS?" when he is supposed to be telling you about your spinal tap results. It may sound like a bad joke, but this was the gentle way my diagnosis was handed to me.

While many people would be angered by such an outrageous slip, I actually appreciated it more than I would have an hour-long "I've got something to tell you Ms. Moorhead please sit down" speech. I was relieved to finally have an explanation for the weird and frightening things happening to my body, the way my balance was off and the room seemed to sway as I walked, the memory and speech problems, and the now-constant tremor of my hands.

This diagnosis, although difficult, was comforting — considering that neurologist #1 had hinted that I was insane. He had asked me why I was slurring my words, and I explained that I had bitten my tongue in my sleep and that my speech sounded funny because my tongue hurt. He asked if I had done this before, and I answered in the affirmative. To this, he wrote in my file, "history of tongue biting." He then ran a neurological exam and pronounced that I was most likely epileptic. One unremarkable EEG later, he pronounced that I needed a shrink. Sobbing and enraged, I went home, recalling stories of how grandpa was a lunatic. I began to cite every panic attack and emotional outburst I had experienced in my life so far as proof that the neurologist might be right.

My biggest fear was that I was losing my mind. I never realized how close to the truth that was. I wasn't losing my mind to insanity but to small lesions or holes in my brain left by an immune system gone berserk. Considering that I could have had lesions on my spine, and that, since my two spinal taps, the image of anything on or in my back made me feel like retching, having holes in my head was just fine. Plus, it didn't even feel like I had holes in my head at all.

The newfound sense of relief that I'd experienced when neurologist #2 slipped up lasted about 20 minutes. My mind began to come up with various dramatic scenes that I just *knew* would be happening to me, from death and wheelchairs to loss of speech and (god forbid), forgetting my PIN number. In that order.

Most people who have little to no knowledge of multiple sclerosis react, I have found, in a similar manner. (Sans running about yelling, "the sky is falling," which only served to panic my husband.) When given the final diagnosis, their instantaneous thought is "How long do I have to live?" followed quickly by "Okay, I'm not going to die but when will I be in a wheelchair?" As I learned more about the condition via books and the Internet, I began to focus my fears on my symptoms: If my speech faltered, would I eventually lose it? If my memory were failing, would it someday be gone? Would I turn into my grandmother who had Alzheimer's, and wander about the house, stashing pens in the bathroom?

By the time we got home from the neurologist's office, my husband was dealing with a babbling basket case who, through sheer willpower, managed not to sob but merely let out the occasional snort in an attempt to "keep it together." We had thought the doctor was looking for MS and, from the information I had gleaned from my computer and books, we expected MS to be the final diagnosis. We were prepared — we thought. Yet when Dr. Jekyll had a Mr. Hyde moment and finally uttered the diagnosis by accident, the tower of strength I expected to be turned out to be more like the wavering tower of nerves.

Considering that my lawyer changed sexes during a case and my mother, who was an assemblywoman, used to get death threats, this turn of events should not have been too shocking. But it was. The shock lay not in the pronouncement of the diagnosis or in the diagnosis itself, but in the realization that I no longer had control of my body.

According to what I'd read, the latest "guess" on the cause of MS was that the white cells, which are primarily the great warriors of your immune system, suddenly decide to stage a coup. These guys begin attacking the myelin — think outer city wall that protects the nerves, the kingdom's workers. When these rogue knights get into the city and begin to wreak havoc on the workers — the nerves themselves — things go berserk.

The brain (or king, as I like to think of it) needs these workers to run the kingdom by sending a series of orderly missives to the land. When the workers are injured or captured, the messages get distorted or completely changed. So when the king (brain) sends out a missive about regulating food supplies (the stomach is full) and the worker (nerve) whose eyesight has not been the same since that last battle, can't read it correctly, the message gets confused. Instead of food supplies being regulated, the worker thinks he's supposed to lay a fire in the main hall to regulate the heat supply, and you suddenly feel as if your body is covered with sunburn.

For most people who have the form of the disease called relapsing/remitting MS, the battle will cease and all will be well in the land again. That period of peace and tranquility is called remission. But, like the clans of Scotland's history, there is always something to fight about. When the argument picks up again and the errant knights once again lay siege to the kingdom, the person will experience a relapse.

For people with progressive MS, it is a constant battle they are bound to lose. While those with relapsing/remitting Multiple Sclerosis have periods of victory in which they are lulled into a sense of peace, the person with progressive MS can only hope that the battle is a long, slow fight and that, by the time things look dim, a cure will be found. The kingdom won't fall, as MS is not fatal, but it can leave the place in disrepair, making a great castle look more like a fragile ruin.

For all types of MS the damage and ruin left behind by the raging rogue army in the brain and spinal cord is in the form of "many scars, or lesions.

So I understood how it had happened. Yet no one could explain to me why it had happened. There was no cure, no reason, and I was no longer in the driver's seat. It's quite a surreal feeling to lie on your bed and *know* that you have holes in your head. It makes for a wonderful excuse any time you do something stupid, but also brings up that eerie childhood fear that your brain just might leak out of your ears. Being the mature individual that I am, I knew this wasn't true, yet I began absently patting my pillow each morning for wet spots.

Not only had I become a passenger in my own body, subjected to its whims and follies, but I also became a passenger in my own car. Neurologist #1 took my description of a brownout-like feeling in my head to mean that I had lapses of consciousness. I imagined this sadist sitting at his desk laughing maniacally while dashing off notes to the DMV. His report of tongue biting and lapses of consciousness caused me to lose the privilege of controlling my own car. It would take me two years to get my license back. The feeling of being a passenger in my own body continued. This is no longer my body, I would think; could those white cells be eating away at my nerves right now? Are they making big holes or small ones? What interesting shapes are they gnawing now?

My first exacerbation, in March of 1999, felt like a car wreck. I found myself returning from what was supposed to have been a two-week trip to London, within 48 hours of arriving. After awakening in the night confused about where I was, walking to the bathroom on weak legs and subsequently losing bladder control, I came home doped up on Valium and frightened for my life (although when doped up on Valium you're actually more interested in napping than in whether you live or die). The exacerbation came out of nowhere. Everything seemed to shatter around me. Yet, though I was battered and in shock, I lived. It took months to regain my strength. During these months my husband and I became more intimate than I ever dreamed possible. He helped me bathe, and he shaved my legs, since I could not keep a grip on the razor.

I spent the next few months on the edge of that passenger seat awaiting the next big crash. The next crash never came. Not a big crash, anyway, but a series of sharp turns, potholes, and near misses throughout each day as I learned my way along the road.

With the same undeniable curiosity that a child has when removing a Band-Aid to pick at a scab, I began to study everything about MS. Like a child I was excited to discover what lay underneath, but afraid of any pain or revulsion I might experience. I wasn't intending to fight it any longer and I wasn't intending to ignore it. I couldn't. I simply had to know what the holes looked like. So books began to pile up, my computer became filled with bookmarks, and I joined the National Multiple Sclerosis Society since it seemed like the thing to do.

What amazed me about the range of MS books was that they all seemed the same. That would imply not much of a "range." I mean, how many different choices must you have to make a "range of choices"? Some books told me all about someone else's diagnosis; others focused on what MS is and how it is diagnosed. My interest began to slide from curiosity about the holes in my head to what a person is supposed to do *after* the diagnosis. Other books went a bit further into how the diagnosis would affect relationships — and stopped there. I was thrilled to discover that anger and disbelief were quite normal, but I was not all that interested in being told by a group of doctors how I would "most likely" feel. Especially when they weren't *in* my body.

The one book I carried about as my bible and still recommend to this day is *Women Living with Multiple Sclerosis* by Judith Lynn Nichols. Her book, which is made up completely of email exchanges between women who have MS, not only gave me the knowledge that others felt the same way I did, but made me laugh. I resolved to laugh at my MS, to thumb my nose at it, and to live my life exactly as I had before. But first, I needed a drink. It was much easier to do my MS research and find it, and my life, hysterically funny, when I couldn't feel my legs.

Chapter 2

Haven't You Heard Yet?

While I drank myself into hysteria, word began to spread about my diagnosis. Soon everyone knew about it. I could walk into a room and tell who had gotten the word by who had suddenly taken an excited interest in the manufacturer of the beige carpet. In my family, whatever one member tells another is pretty much considered a press release. Unless orders are specifically given for the information not to be leaked, everyone hears it as part of our regular updates on each other's life. Even when something is top secret, it tends to slip out under cover of "She can't know you know."

Luckily, I was not overly concerned about keeping my disease to myself, and therefore was not shocked or hurt when I found most people staring at the floor as I entered a room. Since my symptoms were predominantly invisible to the casual onlooker, I was more inclined to wear a sign saying "Got MS" than to hide it. I wanted the world to be aware of my diagnosis by a medical professional; that was my ammo against those who had raised suspicious eyebrows throughout my diagnostic period.

I actually found it kind of amusing that some people apparently couldn't figure out whether it was okay that they knew about my diagnosis and therefore could speak about it freely, or if it was supposed to be some big secret. If they'd heard of my diagnosis from someone else, they tended to be first on the "fascinated with carpet fuzz" list. They seemed so used to finding out about other people's conditions through the grapevine, under pain of death if they uttered a word, that they weren't sure if it was okay to talk about it or not.

Now, if someone has told you that Bob has cancer, and he doesn't mind that people know, you feel able to offer him your support and concern. On the other hand, if someone has told you that Bob has cancer and not verified whether you're supposed to know it, it becomes an uncomfortable situation. You might find yourself avoiding Bob entirely, or nervous that you might accidentally mention cancer in a conversation and then wonder if he knows you know, while *he* wonders if you know, and everyone starts behaving like actors in a bad melodrama:

"I know you know, but are pretending not to know."

"I know you know I am pretending not to know what you know I know."

"But how could you know?"

"The butler told me!" (Insert cheesy organ music here.)

Suddenly, whether or not people knew and how they found out was becoming a problem. Every time I found someone staring at the carpet, I would think, "Okay, does she know? Does she know that I know she knows and that it's okay to know? Or does she think it's not okay to know and is going to avoid any conversation about health so I don't know she knows?"

As far as I'm concerned, it should be common knowledge that Lorna has MS rather than have it become my secret label, solemnly whispered in whichever corner of the family gathering I'm not: "Oh, over there? That's Lorna. *She has MS.*" That kind of secrecy only leads to people frantically trying to avoid you or, possibly even worse, to uncomfortable conversations about floor coverings.

Telling my five-year-old son about my diagnosis was a different story. I didn't know how to explain that I could no longer carry him on my shoulders or play "horse" with him for hours on end. The mommy who had once toted him about on her back and lifted him into the sky over and over like he was a feather had disappeared, and in her place was a lady who spent more time on her butt than on her feet. Knowing that someday my son would notice that not all mothers went about on their butts, I began to ponder when he should be told about my MS. I decided it would be best to share things with him when he was old enough to understand, which I figured might be at about age 9 or 10. This plan was ruined when he came home one day and worriedly asked if I was dying.

After restraining the urge to discover, hunt down, and have on a platter the head of the relative who had planted this destructive thought in my son's mind, I attempted to discover how he came about this idea. From what I could glean from an upset and confused five-year-old, it seemed that he had simply overheard a relative say something about death and me to someone else. Whether it had been told to him directly or not didn't matter; his fear was real.

At the time I was just about Stephan's only playmate, and now all his playmate wanted to do was curl up with her "blankie." Stephan was not convinced that "pet mommy's back while she sleeps" was a real game that every kid just couldn't wait to play. In addition, he had begun to ask questions about why mommy poked herself with a needle every night. So I felt it was time to explain my condition, and its treatment, to him as best I could.

But how would I do that? The answer came while we were watching a movie called *Small Soldiers*, in where good toys were pitted against bad toys. He accepted my explanation that I wasn't dying, simply battling with bad soldiers. I used the same inspired metaphor later, in an article that ran on Mother's Day in a Christian newsletter for those with chronic illnesses, *And He Will Give You Rest* from Rest Ministries.

When I sat Stephan down for the big MS speech, I knew he first needed to understand some basics about the body. I couldn't tell him about a problem with my brain when he didn't know what a brain was. Dragging out some paper and crayons, I hoped that I would be able to ease his fears just a little. Fascinated that mommy was reversing her role and taking out the crayons instead of putting them away; he immediately became enthralled.

First, I drew Mr. Stick Figure. He had a big circle for a head; then I drew a kidney bean shape inside it for his brain. Tracing the brain over and over with my crayon so that Stephan would focus on it, I told him this was the part inside our head that we call a brain. To make this clearer, I took some time to tell him about what other parts we have in our bodies — our heart, our bones, our muscles and so on. Stephan wanted to know how our parts got into our bodies. I began to explain that we were born with our parts, which led to his question "But who put them in?" followed by the matter-of-fact statement "We don't have a lid." This in turn led to a brief but vigorous session of cleaning up the coffee that mommy spit from her mouth when she burst out laughing and went into a sputtering coughing fit.

Thereafter, we dropped the parts procedure and began getting on the nerves. I sketched blue lines from the brain to different parts of the body — the hands, feet, and legs — explaining that these lines were called nerves. I told him that the brain in Mr. Stick's head sent messages or orders through those lines in the body. At this point, my drawing looked like poor Mr. Stick had had a run-in with a jellyfish. These messages, I explained to Stephan, tell Mr. Stick's body what to do. They tell him when to blink, cough, smile, and laugh. My choice of blue for the nerve color led to another sidetrack about whether or not the blue lines he could see under *his* skin were nerves. Feeling completely inadequate at this point and getting a bit fatigued, I told him it was a question for his dad, and attempted to drag him back to our topic.

Drawing from this point (no pun intended), I asked him what he thought would happen if one of those blue lines was blocked when a message was sent down it. The bright five-year-old who could dismantle a complicated toy in 2.5 seconds responded, "things wouldn't move." And, being a smart kid, he probed: "What blocked it?" When I muttered "messed-up myelin," he asked what type of monster Myelin was. I headed for the fridge.

Pulling out a hotdog and hotdog bun, I prayed that Stephan would follow my jump from playing with paper to playing with food, and that God would forgive me should I lose it and run screaming from the room if Stephan found another flaw in my description with which to interrogate me. I was beginning to feel as if I were stuck in a cell with a miniature genius scientist who had to examine every possibility and have every question answered. While I was proud of my son's inquisitiveness, my lack of answers —rather, answers that wouldn't lead to another hundred questions — was beginning to drain my already-damaged brain. I wanted to find a blankie and announce naptime. Now.

Instead, taking a steadying breath, I waved the hotdog and said, "This is the nerve, the line that the messages go down." He said, "Mom, it's a hotdog." I excused myself and went to the bathroom, where I not only cursed a bit but also gently banged my head against the door. Strangling the person who had said the words "dying" and "Lorna" in one sentence — and getting away with it — was looking like an easier task at this point than explaining MS to my son.

Reminding myself that I was the one who had successfully explained to this child how a bathtub worked and why he should not worry that he would be sucked down if he opened the drain, I marched back into the kitchen. We immediately entered into a debate as to whether or not we could pretend that the hotdog was a nerve, followed by a complicated argument about whether or not we had hotdogs in our body. Finally, the MS description moved on.

The bun, I explained was the coating or myelin that protected the "nervedog." After warming the hotdog and popping it into the bun, I asked Stephan whether it looked good to eat. I let him take some bites out of the sides and, after another battle of wills, a chunk out of the middle — not enough to break the hotdog but to make it rather floppy. I was on the verge of explaining how the holes in the bun and the chunks missing from the hotdog were what happened to my nerves, when he said, "But *I* ate the nervedog cover. What eats your covers?"

This is where the *Small Soldiers* movie came in. I explained that in our bodies were white cells that are normally supposed to be soldiers that fight off germs. I explained that some of my soldiers weren't doing what they were supposed to be doing anymore, like the Commandos in the movie. The soldiers had decided they'd rather attack the coatings of the nervedogs than fight germs. The shots I gave myself were good soldiers, like the Gorgonites in the movie that made the bad soldiers stop attacking the nervedogs.

Although what my shots actually did was a bit more complicated than that, my explanation sufficed. My son could comprehend the fact that I was injecting good fighters into my skin to fight the bad guys. Finishing up the hotdog, he seemed comforted by the knowledge that mommy was not being hurt, that my shots and I were winning the war, and I was nowhere near dying. Reminding me to ask daddy about blue nervedogs, he ran off to play "white cell soldier" in the backyard.

I do not profess to know what will happen to my son's psyche because of the way I explained my disease to him. I watched him from the window, wondering if someday I would get a call from some institution where he's strapped up in a room yelling, "KILL ALL WHITE CELLS!" But for now, Mommy was not dying, and that was all that mattered.

In telling my son and others about my MS, I have learned that when it comes to these "invisible" conditions, telling is never as difficult as getting someone to understand. If I took the lead and acknowledged my own condition, people would relax, and the first hurdle of "telling" would be cleared. No matter how silly I felt asking "Have you heard about my MS?" – which sounded comparable to asking, "Have you heard about my rash?" — it worked to lift a person's eye from the carpet to my face.

I wished this simple encouragement on my part would have magically made everyone comfortable with and adjusted to my condition, but it didn't. It seemed that finding out about my Multiple Sclerosis was only the first stage of an odd and sometimes hurtful process of acceptance.

CHAPTER 3

"But You Look So Good"

Most of us have been taught by our parents that "if you can't say something nice, don't say anything at all." This rule bends a bit as we get older, becoming "if you can't say something nice, lie." Case in point: "You don't look fat." So it's not surprising that, when faced with a loved one who has MS, the first thing to spill from a person's lips is a compliment such as "you look so good."

I have no problem with the "look so good" opening; what bothers me is the "look so good" response. The "look so good" response always begins with a friend or loved one asking "How are you doing?" Whether answered with the truth — "Due to bladder problems and fatigue, I'm thinking of getting a bed pan; I wonder if they come in purple" — or the path of least resistance, simply a mumbled "fine," the punch line is always the same: "But you look so good." Or worse, "Well, it doesn't seem to be affecting you that much." (How much is "much"? Was there a "much" requirement that I wasn't told about?) The pain and anger unintentionally inflicted on me by those "you look so good" responses reminded me of the joke in which an animal is run over twice, once by accident and a second time as the idiot driver backs up to see what he hit.

I suppose my friends and loved ones intended to pep me up. But I felt like one of those miserable old guys who keep hearing "at least you still have your health." What the heck did people expect I was going to say to this? "Wow, you know you're right; so what if I can't play "horsey" with my son anymore, or dance, or balance my check book, or use knives safely, but hey, I look damn good and that's all that matters! Thanks for reminding me!" I would rather have someone ask a dumb question about my condition — for example, "When are you starting chemotherapy?" — than ask me how I was feeling and then dismiss whatever I told them with "but you look great!"

If it weren't so socially unacceptable I would have slapped each person upside the head each time they made that comment. I began to wonder if phrases like "You don't look sick" or "But you look so good" had been recommended in a book called *How To React Politely to A Loved One's Disease*. I imagined that the chapter on "How to respond when the person complains about their disease" would include a passage like this:

In the event that you ask how the person is feeling and they actually tell you, always remind them of how good they look, or tell them they do not look sick. Such statements will keep the person calmer and less depressed. Your lying plays an important role in helping them avoid needless acknowledgement of their illness. Keep in mind, also, that if the person doesn't appear ill, he or she may be faking

Now correct me if I am wrong, but isn't lying supposed to be a bad thing? Aren't we supposed to get angry and ground someone when they lie to us? Since when did it become a good thing to lie to someone? (I really need the info on this because there are many instances of lying in my childhood and I could get my sentences dropped if this turns out to be some loop-hole in my defense. Besides my five-year-old son should be hitting the "lying about the broken vase" age any day now.)

Whether people made this comment because they were uncomfortable hearing the truth about how I was doing, or because they thought it was helpful, it still gave the impression that, to them, I couldn't be *that* sick. So if I didn't appear *that* sick, maybe I wasn't *sick* at all. It wasn't just my little deluded brain coming up with this line of reasoning. Members of the public displayed it more often than not.

One summer day a police officer approached me after my husband and I parked in the handicap spot. I looked "too good" in my sundress and sandals, and he questioned whether I had the right to be there. While he called in the placard number, I sat in a hot car feeling not only embarrassed and angry, but miserable as well. Heat and stress often cause the average daily MS symptoms to worsen. For me this meant my fatigue worsened, I found it increasingly harder to think, and my usual small hand and arm tremors became a visible shaking.

After he received the reply on his radio that yes, Lorna Moorhead had been issued a handicap placard, the officer left. No apology, no "Gee, I'm a insensitive jerk for thinking that just because you look young and healthy, you can't have a disability. I guess I really am a pig." I would have taken his badge number and started a crusade using the Americans with Disabilities Act as my springboard, if I hadn't needed a nap so badly.

Episodes like that only helped to increase my suspicion that when people said, "you look good" they were really saying "You look good, so you really can't be all that sick." When I spoke to other MSers via the Internet, they too talked of this type of discrimination. I suddenly realized that for those of us with invisible symptoms came the stigma of "looking good." For the first time in my life I really got a taste of what it felt like to be discriminated against, to have someone instantly dislike you for the way you look. People like that policeman were not the only ones who displayed discrimination. In the year that followed my dx, my car was keyed, its antenna broken, and I got accusing looks and comments – from other disabled people. I became afraid to use the handicap parking spot and other privileges that I was completely entitled to. All because I looked "so good."

My MS became a silent partner. Always there, wrapped about me like a lover, but completely hidden to everyone who looked at me. At this point, a year after my first symptom and only a month after my final dx, I would have given anything to have someone notice the tremors in my hands, my slow walk, and the pauses in my speech as I tried in vain to think of a word like "chicken." I prayed that someone would take the time to see my symptoms, acknowledge them, and face them with me. But the grocery store clerk thought I was drunk, another person took my pauses to mean I was finished speaking, and of course my tremors must have been from too much coffee.

I was confident, though, that I wouldn't encounter this "look so good = not that sick" bias within the medical profession. Surely my primary care physician and my neurologist would see the debilitating fatigue in my eyes, hear the slur of my words, and notice the change in my gait. Yeah, right. Considering that neurologist #1 had told me to see a shrink, my spinal fluid had been lost by the Keystone Cops dressed up as lab technicians — causing me to have not one but two delightful spinal taps in the course of the diagnostic process — and my diagnosis had been blurted out by accident weeks before it became final, I should not have been so damn surprised.

Yet I had good memories of the medical profession, too — of the pediatrician who gave me lollipops, the obstetrician who delivered my son, and neurologist #2 who fought for my diagnosis when others thought I was crazy. I struggled between these shining examples of health care and the cold truth: Medicine is about as bipolar as Henry VIII when it comes to care of patients. One minute they love you, the next — off with your head. These people were faster with the "you look good" phrase than grandma with a duster. (And she was a mad duster. From 0 to dusted in about 2.5 seconds.)

It is hurtful to feel that a friend has told you "you look good" because they cannot really see your illness, but it is devastating to have your doctor say it. This person is in charge of your care. If they don't think you're suffering, how will you get help? This is what led me to one of my MS rules: Don't always wear makeup to the doctor's office. This definitely applies to the men, unless they want to see a psychologist who will most likely tell them they "look good" and ask about their grandmother's dusting habits.

Why would someone, let alone a doctor, be so distracted by looks? I was enraged that anyone would make presumptions about my health based on my appearance. My husband was the first to play devil's advocate. As I lay on the bed, collapsed in fatigue and yelling at the ceiling about insensitive, uncaring people, he interjected, "Hon, you spent an hour doing your hair and makeup this morning. Surely a person who can take the time to do all that is feeling good." Pausing in mid-rant, I glared at him. He merely shrugged and said, "Think about it. Remember when your parents would say 'if you're well enough to play, you're well enough to go to school'? The same thing applies here." By God, he made sense. What a brilliant observation about why doctors, and loved ones for that matter, might be thinking I was fine.

I was irritated by his insight as only a woman out-thought by a man can be. I decided to prove him wrong. I would do an experiment. I went to my next doctor's appointment dressed nicely, with my hair and face done, and to the one after that in more comfortable clothes with no makeup on. During which visit do you think I made the most progress? Do I really have to tell you? On the first visit, her response to my complaints was "Well, you look good." On the second, she said nothing about "looking good" and I got a prescription for one of my symptoms.

Still following the scientific method, I believed that perhaps this phenomenon was limited to one health professional, and tried the experiment on another. The same thing happened. During the first visit I was consoled with how great I looked and sent on my way with nothing but "call if you feel worse." The second time I was actually examined and a test was ordered. This happened not only with doctors, but also with psychologists, friends, and the lady at the camera counter. One day, dressed up, I was "looking good," the next, it was "you look tired, sweetheart."

The point was never to make myself look sick, but to not go out of my way to make myself look "fine." When people saw Lorna with her hair curled, her makeup on, sitting calmly in a chair, they had no way of knowing that the ground felt like it was moving under me, I wanted nothing more than to fall asleep, and I was having trouble following the conversation. They had no way of knowing that my hands were folded in my lap to keep them from shaking. That my legs were crossed to keep them from twitching. A doctor or loved one does not have the ability to jump into my skin and know how I'm truly feeling. They can't see through my eyes; it was unfair of me to expect them to. So I decided that, when I was really having a problem that I did not want to be overlooked, I would not go out of my way to look "presentable."

But I'm still a proud woman, so I take my makeup in the

CHAPTER 4

The Peanut Gallery:
Friends, Family, and Everyone In-between

My extended family always made it a priority to get together for family events and holidays. During holiday dinners I recall a statement that came up quite often: "We're so lucky as a family. We've never lost anyone to a tragedy such as a car accident. No one has been struck down with a terrible illness or disability. We're so lucky. Thank God for that." We would raise our glasses and knock on wood. Each year it amazed and fascinated me that these statements were true. A family of 5 siblings had never been hit hard by the unpredictable tragedies of life. Often after my diagnosis I wondered if anybody thought, should we of knocked on wood more often? Did we somehow curse ourselves by being thankful?

Sure, when it came to minor dramas I was usually center stage, but no one, (including almost all my friends) had ever experienced major trauma. Unfortunately for me there seemed to be an issue with typecasting. My life thus far had followed like a bad drama (with a lot of good luck), getting accepted and dropping out of two prestigious schools, pregnant, married, and divorced in only four years. Many relatives in reaction to my diagnosis seemed to decide that, considering my hectic life, I could "handle anything thrown at me." The idea that "this always happens to Lorna" still plagues me.

So while my illness was tragic, it also came off like a soap opera campaign to gain ratings. I could envision a group of scriptwriters sitting around a huge table saying: "*People haven't been watching Days of Lorna's Life. We need to raise ratings- Hey I know let's give her a tragic illness!*" My family's reaction to my illness was the same as it had been when I left a school or got divorced: Give Lorna a pep talk and sooner or later she'll get it together. I felt like the boy who cried wolf.

While the prevailing sentiment was that I would eventually "buck up" and handle the MS dx fine, my relationships began to change. Even my relationship with the garbage man changed from anonymity to tense discussions about why the can wasn't all the way down the drive like it should be. Most MS books warn a person about this. (About relationship changes not the obtuse behavior of one's gabrage man.) But while the books made this transformation sound as obvious and colorful as Dorothy's first glance of Oz, in real life the changes came about in shades of gray.

Speaking of change, while my father most likely felt powerless since I hit puberty, my mother had always been able to single handedly fix anything I threw her way. (This amazing ability to handle not only my crises but also those of 4 other children was one of the reasons I nicknamed her the Matriarchal Octopus.) Everyone knows that parents have the answer to everything and mothers in particular can make anything better. Got a cold? Mom has the right old-fashioned remedy. Unhappy with being in high school? Mom can show you how to use what you've learned to get through. Sure she lost her grip some when I became pregnant at 19, (*You're WHAT?!?*) but within months she was back offering books and wisdom like "Leave some crackers by your bed to ease the morning sickness."

However, Multiple Sclerosis was not something in Mom's Mary Poppins bag of sugar solutions and we both knew it. After all those times when I would get sick or unravel in front of her, I now found myself nervous about showing how I felt. I didn't want to whine and I didn't want her to feel bad. After all this was the first illness of mine that she could not fix, and it must be tearing her apart. Therefore, at her house on Thanksgiving and the third month after my dx, when I woke up only to fall down with my legs not working, I sat on the floor debating whether to call for her help or keep it to myself.

After rubbing my legs vigorously hoping to "wake them up", it became obvious to me that while I had feeling in them they were not going to hold my weight. So I used my arms to roll over and began to crawl to the bedroom door. As I made my way across the hall, I felt horrible and thought I must look like I was imitating some army recruit squirming under barbed wire. Being in such an unbelievable position, I felt like Mom might think I was faking. After all it was the holidays and I *was* the drama queen. As got to the foot of the stairs, I saw my stepfather, Gordon, in the office in front of me look over. He gave me an odd grin as if to say, "What are you up to now?"

Embarrassed and in what must have been shock, I replied in an overly animated voice, "My legs aren't working right."(I sounded down right chipper.) My stepfather noted that he had heard an awfully loud banging sound only a minute before however, he had figured the bed had broken or something. The idea that at 23 I was still breaking beds, went to show how well adjusted my family was to "Lorna catastrophes". Just when I was getting ready to ask him how in God's name he thought I had gone about breaking my bed, my mother shouted down from her bedroom "WHAT happened?"

I knew she'd been listening. When I was about 7 my mother informed me that not only did mothers have eyes in the backs of their heads, but also they could hear like bats. I knew she would have her ears cocked toward the stairs as soon as I began to inform Gordon of my plight.

"I fell down. My legs aren't working right." I called back up the stairs. I moved to sit on the stairs, and my mother rushed to the top of the stairs obviously worried.

"You fell? Where? Are you okay? Do you need a doctor? What do you need?" Looking up at my mother's concerned face from my position on the stairs seemed very much like a scene that should of played when I was a child. After all adults don't go falling out of bed and crawling about the halls.

"My knees hurt a bit and my legs feel like jelly. But I think I'm fine. The sensation is coming back, I just can't stand on them." Since my mother lived in a small coastal town and I knew there was no emergency room within miles, I attempted to keep myself from emotionally falling apart. I focused on how to simply get through the rest of the day without being too much of a nuisance.

"I don't think I need a doctor as the feeling is coming back. I probably just pushed myself too far yesterday, with all the walking. Could I have some help to the bathroom so I can take a bath? I don't think I can stand for a shower." I felt completely unworthy of asking for help. Along with this feeling came a strong urge to downplay the shocking situation as much as I possibly could. With my husband I had become almost at ease with my MS problems but with my mother I felt like I shouldn't have this much control over a situation, like a kid playing hooky. For some reason the idea of me telling my mother what I needed, being the one to give orders about my own health seemed wrong. Mom was supposed to tell me what I needed to do. That was the way it had always been. But she couldn't.

Mom simply smiled and came down the stairs to help me into the bathroom. While I took my bath she checked on me and I kept shooing her off with a half-smile and "I'm fine", so that she could focus on cooking and preparing for the guests who were to be arriving. While I sat in the tub staring down at my legs and holding back absolute fear, I fretted about ruining a family holiday with my MS. I simply wished I could disappear.

I soon got enough feeling and strength back into my legs to stand for short periods, like shifting from the ground to a chair, which Mom had brought in, so I could finish getting ready. While I did my make-up, my mother continued to check in on me, smiling kindly and offering sympathetic words. Each time, I did not respond by being consoled but by feeling guilty. I knew she couldn't make me better and I felt that I was simply adding to her Thanksgiving stress by making her worry. Although I was attempting to avoid any real reaction to what had just happened to me, thoughts raced through my head as I stared at my face in the mirror. *Why is this happening to me? Why did this have to happen now? I've been taking my shots, why are my legs giving out? I can't even control my legs.* The next time my mother came in I was already crying.

Oddly enough she didn't seem surprised, just sad. She held me while I broke into sobs about not having control over my own body. I apologized more than once for burdening her to which she always firmly replied that I wasn't. She asked me questions about what I thought had happened and what my doctor back home could do about it, but could offer no solution. Instead of the old days where Mom always knew in a pinch what was needed, that day I had to swallow my pride, and tell her what I needed. I would've much rather just had her take over and tell me what to do, but things were different now. In this arena only I knew what I needed. We found a nice hiking stick to use as a cane, and nobody seemed to mind that I spent more time sitting on the floor with the grandkids than standing around with adults.

It was on that day that I began to come to terms with our new relationship. This was a subject on which my mother could not "parent" in the sense of fixing it. She could be my friend and read MS books right along side of me, but she would never know exactly what was best for me in any MS-related situation. While she seemed well aware of her new role and took it on without any complaints, it took me being helpless for me to see this change. Unlike my childhood, if I didn't speak up and tell her what I needed, she wasn't going to be able to just psychically "know" and do it. She could stand by me and love me, but she couldn't fix me.

Over the year this relationship developed it's new boundaries. Mom never showed me her sorrow because she didn't wish to add to my pain and I never told her exactly everything about my MS in an attempt to lessen hers. So from a girl who used to seek out her mother in order to "show" her an illness, I now preferred to merely speak about it. When it came to help, if I didn't ask for it, it was assumed it wasn't needed. This wasn't because my family didn't wish to help, but because they didn't know when or how to. I was beginning to learn how to ask for help and it was a rather humbling process.

My parent's relationship changes and reactions were rather painless compared to unpredictable and varying response from everyone else. I think this stems from the idea that our parents have clemency by way of title to make more mistakes. When you become an adult, and realize your parents aren't perfect, you forgive them for showing your naked baby pictures and expect many more embarrassing situations. Friends and siblings are a bit different. As most of us with siblings know it's an unwritten rule that siblings can choose to dislike each other at any given time. Feelings can change as fast as the seasons. I believe that while we love our parents no matter how many flaws they have, (like thinking black socks with flip-flops are great footwear); we seem to hold our siblings and friends to theirs. Brothers and sisters are more closely entwined with love and anger than parents ever are. Friends and siblings are people we choose to be around, not people we have to be around. So while it may be easy to pass off a parent's uncomfortable reactions, a friend's is much harder to ignore.

Such was the case of an old friend of mine whose first question when he found out about my MS was "How long do you have to live?" Regardless of the fact that MS is not terminal, I knew that if I had been dying he would of still asked the same blunt question. So, okay, I passed off that question as a bit rough, but acknowledged that at least he was being open with me. After telling him I was not going to die, he continued to talk and I wished that he hadn't.

He began to tell me how much he missed his dead grandmother! I waited patiently for him to redirect his comments back to my non-deadly condition and away from his deceased relative, but he kept on. I heard about how she died, how much she meant to him, her name, and what she looked like. I merely gripped the armchair so as not to disgrace the memory of his grandmother. Multiple Sclerosis never came up again.

On the other side of this coin were the siblings and friends who cut out every article they could find on MS. These thoughtful gestures were appreciated but sometimes became a bit amusing. There are so many articles, web sites, and "cures" out there that it is hard for my friends to not inform me about them. But magnetic waves causing my MS due to the incorrect placement of my bed? Did they even read the article before they gave it to me? I had so many tapes, phone numbers and addresses that I was filled with a sense of joy for those who were looking out for me, and a sense of humor when confronted with "cures" that were akin to snake oil. I learned to not be offended by these odd bits of information but to simply smile and relish the fact that the person had taken the time to think about helping me.

In the middle of this spectrum with people centered on their own demise on one end and avid article clippers on the other, was the attempt to pass off my MS as no big thing. They would listen to one of my symptom complaints and say, "Well, that happens to me all the time!" This is when I'd usually interject "Yes, but you're over 60 and I'm 23." Another favorite was "I know someone with MS who jogs." *(Who is that person? I've heard them mentioned now by my doctor, friends, and acquaintances. Is this one person or an MS jogging team?)* I believe deep down that these people were trying to make me feel better by attempting to downplay my condition. Yet these comments always left me to wondering: Was I sounding like a hypochondriac? Should I not attempt to share my thoughts on my MS with anyone but my spouse?

There is a fine line between allowing people to recognize your illness and shoving it down their throats. But in attempting to find out where the line was drawn I came up empty handed. I checked all of my beloved web site and MS books to find the answer of how much to share and how much to keep quiet and came up with nothing. In the end I found, the reason there is no definite answer on how to deal with a person's reaction or how much of your condition to show them, is because it changes with each person.

Some remind me of a Sergeant saying something akin to *"So YOU'VE got MS? I stood on top of a hill covered in mines, one leg half off, no back up, AND jock itch! You can't let a little MS get in your way! Lots of people have MS, and they never let it stop them! Why I've have a one legged friend with MS who jogs!"* Ever the optimist this person attempts to make my MS not such a big thing in order to make me feel better. Others are like Counselors who say *"Oh you have MS? How does Lorna feel about that? Is Lorna coping?"* On the darker side there are those who appear like a Movie Star focused on taking center stage *"Oh you have MS? I have gout! And a bad back. Plus I have this lump, do you think I should see a doctor?"*

This also led me to coin a phrase that I call Illness Poker. The Poker game is where one person states a complaint and the other person responds by stating a complaint of theirs that is worse, thereby raising the pot. I would say something like this: "Gosh my

MS is bugging me. My hands seem to have tremors all the time now." Then my loved one would reply: "Really? I have bad arthritis and can barely use my hands. Plus my head is killing me today." (I always could hear in my mind "And I'll raise you a headache.")

Often I would find myself doing this with my husband or one of my parents. Most likely this will come up for me when I am talking to people who are older and more likely to have similar complaints about various body parts. When I mentioned this feeling of being "one upped" by someone when I entered into a discussion about symptoms to my husband, Mark, he admitted that he did it to show his ability to understand my problems. For example that by saying they have arthritis they are not stating that their condition is worse but that they can understand having hand problems. I had never looked at the poker game as a way to express sympathy but once I began to pay attention I found that I did it to my friends! Someone would tell me about a bad experience and I would attempt to let him or her know I understood by relating a bad experience of mine! Once Mark pointed this out I was able to understand why a person said what they did when I talked about my MS and avoided more hurt feelings.

There is a vast array of reactions for every type of person. There are Morticians who ask if you have everything "arranged" for when it's time, the Scientist who asks if you're sure it's MS and have they run the test involving rat spinal cords yet? The Skeptics who think MS is a ruse created by the government, and finally the best type: The Mutts. They are a mixture of the best of each type, who curiously ask you everything about the condition and cry when you cry.

If these different reactions were not confusing enough for the person with MS, the fact that people can change roles is. Some days my mother would be the Sergeant and others a Mutt. But that is all part of my loved ones reaction to MS. It changes as fast as my condition does. There are days when I feel great and days when I feel like the world is coming to an end. Just the same there are days when my family and friends are going to be right there, battling the condition along side me, and others when they are tired of me being sick and tired.

CHAPTER 5

Compensation for Lost Parts

A few months into the first year after my dx of Multiple Sclerosis, I became aware that makeup was not the only way to hide my disability from those around me. As my tremors, sense of distance, and balance got worse; I had begun to subconsciously adapt to them, adjusting my movement, speech, and grip.

While some compensation is necessary in the life of a person with MS, such as using the handicapped spot to conserve walking energy, others can hinder the person by causing extra strain and fatigue on the brain and body. When these "extra" compensations were brought to my attention by my father, after a party which had all but exhausted me, it began an internal struggle about how easy it was to wipe off make-up when I wanted people to recognize my MS and how difficult it was for me to use a cane rather than adjust my gait, so that people would *see* my MS. My legs still worked most of the time, and being a bit off balance does not qualify for the use of a cane. Right?

Therefore, when it came time to attend that party at a fancy restaurant for my stepfather' s 75th birthday, I wore not only makeup but high heels as well. I did not think heels would cause any problems for me, since I *knew* my previous trips and falls were caused by my sons' toys, my dog, and my husband. Everything but my MS.

Contrary to my delusions of stability when I got dressed, at the party I felt as if I were standing on the deck of a rolling ship.

Wearing heels, no less. Because my peripheral vision had a habit of making things look like they were swimming, I compensated not by taking off my shoes or sitting down like any sane person would, but by standing like a sailor with my feet set wide apart. Not the epitome of lady-like, but useful under the circumstances. While standing bow-legged, I gripped my wineglass in both hands, suddenly afraid that with my tremors I would spill it, or drop it and cause a scene. Walking made the rocking worse, so a trip to the bathroom involved more planning and effort than standing with a wine glass.

Weeks earlier at the grocery store, I had learned that looking to the left or right while attempting to walk in a straight line caused me to veer in that direction. I started to compensate by looking straight down and shuffling my feet as I walked. That way I could spy any objects in my path and not veer off the left or right when my head turned that way. Yet now, on the good ship MS, my high heels didn't allow me to shuffle. So, as the true sailor I was, I swaggered to the bathroom shifting my weight from one foot to the other. I felt as if everyone would notice my odd movements and think I was drunk. Not a single eye batted and no one asked if I needed assistance. I *knew* they thought I was drunk.

That night I compensated, making up for lost parts, beautifully. Standing around like a tomboy in her first dress and plotting every step of my long walk to the bathroom, I still wasn't aware how exhausting these compensations could be. I only knew I was simply trying to avoid falling down or causing a catastrophe. Some failing parts seemed to compensate for themselves; as I made subconscious adjustments, things I never really *"thought"* about doing, I just *did*.

For example, how I learned to eat without incident. After what turned out to be, thankfully, an uneventful trip across an ocean of red tile to the bathroom, it was time to eat. I was grateful for the ability to sit, and finally, to eat, since I had forgone the hors d'oeuvres to hold my wineglass. Since tremors had been my first real MS symptom, I had begun compensating for them almost a year before my diagnosis. During that year I unknowingly began to grip my eating and writing utensils tighter in order to control them. At the party I did not really understand the lengths to which I had gone to "cover up" my difficulties until they were pointed out to me later, by my father and Mark.

While I did not always focus on my grip, I *did* focus on my speech. I quickly learned that I could cover long pauses while I searched for a simple word by shoving food in my face. By the time I was finished chewing, my slow brain would usually have found the right word. So I got through dinner this way: gripping the fork as if it were a slippery fish, getting food into my mouth, and thinking about the next witty remark to make to the person on the left while chewing. (And praying to God that I wouldn't suddenly "forget" how to swallow like I had on many occasions before.)

Despite my feeling that everyone, especially my family, would notice these little changes in gait and speech, my compensations did their job. Not a single person noticed, and they told me I looked beautiful. At first I was happy to have pulled it off. In addition, I swore I would never wear heels again. Well, not unless the situation *really* called for them. Nevertheless, two days later I was still exhausted and a tiny feeling of anger had begun to boil deep within my belly. How could they not see how hard it was to wear those damn shoes? Didn't they notice me staggering to and from the bathroom? *Were they blind?!?!*

So I mentioned – okay, I moaned — days later to my father that I did not understand how I could still be so exhausted from simply "sitting pretty" at a party and how frustrated I was that no one had noticed the effort it took me to walk and to speak. In response he asked, "How many things did you do to compensate for your MS? How many things did you do to make sure you didn't fall over or drop something and cause a scene?" I began to count. My husband, who had also become my chauffeur at this point, merely sat back and smiled.

First, I recalled, there was holding on to the wineglass with both hands for fear of dropping it. Second came gliding around the room in heels without actually gliding *into* anything. Third came the act of simply standing while talking and holding the wineglass. Fourth was attempting to speak between bites as quickly and accurately as possible without falling into a long pause.

After I reviewed the conscious compensations I'd made, my father said, "Now tell me about the ones you're not thinking about." I looked at him blankly, wondering if this was a trick question. How could I tell him about what I wasn't thinking about? "Since your first tremors back in August of '98, what things have you done to make sure you don't make a "fool", as you like to say, of yourself?" I began to glower at him, thinking of my dropped coffee cups and my lost footings in the bathtub. Mark took my silence as a cue for him to speak, and softly added "Do you realize that on a day when your tremors are bad, if you attempt to hold your cup with one hand, you grip it so hard your knuckles turn white?" Now, it was my turn to stare at my husband. I already knew I had decided to hold my wineglass with both hands so I wouldn't make a scene at the party, but I had never consciously focused on how tightly I was holding on to things at home. In response, I loosened my grip on the cup I was holding and then put it down when it began to wobble. I waved my hand in dismissal. "I'll admit that I might do that, but those are small things. They shouldn't make me feel this way." I retorted. "How can anyone honestly say that talking, standing, and drinking is hard for them?"

After remarking that it depends on how much you've had to drink, my father said: "You're not *anyone*, Lorna. *You* have MS. Until *you* realize that, number one, you have difficulties caused by *your disability*, and number two, you're only hiding them with these compensations — and these compensations take extra effort — you're going to feel horrible after every engagement."

"Not to mention guilty because you think there's no reason for you to be so tired," my husband chimed in. Here I was with the two men who saw my disabilities clearly and suddenly all I wanted to do was prove them wrong. I was fine. Shuffling my feet to walk and holding my coffee cup with white knuckles were easy tasks. They did not drain me. If they did, that would mean my only solution was to find ways to compensate by appropriate means, like using thick-handled utensils and… a cane. And while I believed I needed to use the handicap spot to shorten my walking time so I wasn't exhausted after shopping trips, I did not feel that I qualified for a cane. It was almost as if I felt, that because I could still use my legs most of the time and compensate by shuffling, I didn't have the *right* to use a cane. *(Besides people would just stare at the young girl with a cane and think she was a fake and I had enough issues already.)*

"The grocery store is hardly an engagement." I blurted out in an attempt to divert where they were going with this. Suddenly, I began to wonder why I wanted everyone to acknowledge my MS yet not *see* the difficulties it caused.

As if reading my mind my father said, "Every time, be it at a party or the grocery store, that you compensate and essentially attempt to hide your difficulties instead of using items such as a cane to assist you, you're going to get tired. You have no one but yourself to blame when people tell you you're doing great. Remember: You're only as true to yourself as you are to your MS."

Great. My father was spouting lines that sounded like they came from a book entitled *More Quotes from Forrest Gump*. I looked to see if Mark was following this and saw that he was pretending to read the newspaper. I could tell by the way his lips twitched that he found this statement highly amusing. Knowing that my father was not going to let up until I acknowledged the sense he was making, and that Mark, who was grinning behind the newspaper was not going to take my side, I merely nodded at my father's words and dropped the subject.

Yet my father had a point. A few points actually. The first was that I had adopted certain habits to counterbalance areas where I was beginning to falter. The second was identifying subconscious actions — like running my hand over the backs of chairs as I passed in case I began to wobble — that developed during a year of trying to "manage" my symptoms while I was being diagnosed. These cover-ups, while not necessarily noticed, were still exhausting to my mind and body. And finally, these cover-ups were essentially that: cover-ups, hiding the everyday difficulties I had from everyone but these two men. This only served to back up the stigma of "looking good", because I *did* look good. I looked just fine. I was choosing to hide my problems with compensations instead of accepting and finding ways to assist them. Attempting to appear "together" when I wasn't, for the sake of pride, was lying. Although saying, "you're only as true to yourself as you are to your MS," sounded hokey, it sounded sort of Zen as well.

But I wasn't willing to listen that day. Sure, I knew my father had made some good points, and was secretly impressed that Mark noticed small things like white knuckles, but I still firmly believed I didn't need *that* type of assistance. It was as if I had fallen prey to the "look too good" statement and believed that I was doing "too well" to need anything like a cane. Firmly believing that I wasn't *that* off-balance, I went on with life. In the weeks to come, my close relationship to door jams and my general lack of balance began to resemble slapstick routines.

In fact, these routines involved what I eventually called the "set up". The "set up" is a quirky little dance in which I lose my grip on an item, dropping it directly in my path so that I can then step on it and forfeit my footing. My compensations became more exhausting as I began to rely on them more and more, especially when it came to balance. I found myself more often than not, thinking my way technically across each room. I would approach a situation feeling more like a programmer than a woman. *"Now I'm going to slow down, then shift to the right to get past the couch, and circle the coffee table. Should any pets or children block the way, I'm going to shut down the system momentarily, reprogram, and restart. Do not attempt to step over roadblock as it will cause a system failure which will lead to a system crash."*

These compensations for my lack of depth perception and balance were unfortunately hardly noticeable to anyone other than my father and husband. (As my other family members would of insisted I get a cane if they had known how in-depth my walking plans had become.) The average person most likely assumed I stared at the floor when I walked because I had low self-esteem, not because I was looking out for roadblocks. This penchant for flailing about a room was heartbreaking. *(For a woman who took ballet at age 4, musical theater from 14 to 16, and thrived on the dance club scene at 18, I'd rather it be assumed I was having a spaz moment than thought that my grace was gone forever due to disability.)*

As the MS performances came more frequently, I continued to pass off the entire routine as simply coincidence or bad timing, and always vowed to watch my step closer next time. *Because only people who have really bad legs all the time and appear ill can use canes. Besides, using a cane will only slow me down and cause more problems.* This inner-critic which spoke up every time I thought of getting a cane, helped complicate the war between the part of me that believed I needed help (and became indignant when people told me how great I was doing) and the part that felt I was too healthy for real help.

I did begin to notice however, that I could tell whether a day was going to be good or bad, MS-wise, by how many things I crashed into that morning. If I could get dressed without major incident I had a fair chance at a good day. Most days *Major Incident* seemed like my stage name. I imagined a ballet program that read:

> Act 1. Slam shoulder into doorframe on way out of bathroom. Step on son's toy. Lift foot in pain and lose balance.
> Act 2. Try to take step forward to regain balance. Stub toe on bed.
> Finale: Fall onto bed.

At the end of the month and many spills after that conversation with my father, I found myself lying on my lawn with a twisted ankle. My husband had already installed a handrail in the shower, with a minor bit of grousing on my part, but this time was not home to save me. I was far enough out in our large backyard that Stephan, who was in the house, could not hear me. I had never twisted an ankle in my life. Well, except for when I was about 10 but that involved roller skates and doesn't count. Ladies as graceful as I didn't go about bumping into things and tripping over their feet. I stared at the ground in pain and near tears with two voices raging in my head. *Give it up Lorna, you've got balance problems and should get a cane. You don't have to use it all the time, just on those mornings when you feel wobbly. Shuffling your feet is obviously not solving the problem.* And then the critic: *Oh come on! Your legs work and you know how silly a young lady like yourself is going to look with a cane. You know everyone will think you don't need it and you're just a big drama queen, like they always have. You just need to pay more attention to where you're going!* So there I was highly frustrated with myself for falling again, tears running down my cheeks, and calling my dog to see if, with a moment's coaching, he could do a Lassie and "go get help." The dog, as close to Lassie as I was to Ginger Rogers at the moment, went into the house to eat.

While I sat on the cold lawn with the morning dew soaking into my pants, I retraced my steps in my mind to decide where I had gone wrong this time. I knew I had gone outside for something important. Of that I was sure, because it was winter and I usually didn't go ambling about in the cold unless I REALLY had to. At this point, due to emotional stress and a knack for cognitive problems with my MS, I couldn't tell you what I had ventured out for, but I was sure this essential item, was in the backyard. The next thing I knew, I had fallen on the grass and when I attempted to stand again, my ankle surged with pain. Even the dog had looked at me in shock. He had loped closer, staring at me and then at the ground, devoid of any objects that could have caused my fall, then back at me as if to say "Why'd you throw yourself on the ground?" I was sure that from that moment on the border collie was going to regard me as not only lacking in the ability to throw a Frisbee far enough, but wanting in the gravity department as well.

While most people would have passed off this little incident as simply "tripping over one's feet." For me it was the point where I conceded that my recent series of slapstick routines were *not* temporary bouts of clumsiness but the opening act for mishaps to come. As I crawled on my hands and knees toward the house, hoping the neighbors didn't see, the critic in my head began to loose its argument to my own common sense. I felt a bit ashamed at my behavior and very silly for letting myself go this far. I was the epitome of a hypocrite expecting people to notice my MS all the while not using the assistance I needed because I worried how it would make me look.

Maybe it was because this time I had actually injured myself, but it finally sank in that my bumping, dropping, and falling spells were *not* going away, and that all my compensations, while they might be temporarily useful for making me look wonderfully unaffected at parties, weren't truly helping. These slapstick routines were "choreographed by MonSter," not by chance. It was time I faced the music, so to speak, and realized that my new life's soundtrack was closer to "Looney Tunes" than "Flashdance".

When Christmas arrived days later, my husband, who had been silently waiting for the big fall that would wake me up, presented me with a beautiful cane. I smiled at the shiny blue swirls on it and fought back one last urge to scream, "I'm fine. I don't need this. It was an accident!" Because I wasn't fine. He had seen the bruises, scrapes, and finally the twisted ankle. So at Christmas, he not only gave me a cane, but a choice. I could acknowledge my disability and use my cane with pride, or I could continue painfully compensating for lost parts.

CHAPTER 6

Not Tonight Dear, I Have MS

When they talked about sexual problems in MS, I always thought they were talking about the men. In fact most of the books I read devoted their section on sex to the problems a man might face. So I never thought that my disease would interfere with that area of my life. *(I should have seen it coming.)* MS had already intruded upon my ability to be supermom; why leave my status of love goddess alone?

Once again I had made the mistake of underestimating my adversary. I have since learned that just because the books don't address it, doesn't mean MS can't do it. MS is a bit like God this way. It seems able to create anything it wants whenever it feels like it. God wants a chicken, he gets a chicken, MS wants to give you an odd feeling in your left foot, it can.

There came a time about six months after my diagnosis when I just didn't want to have sex anymore. I was constantly fatigued, my skin and muscles had become so sensitive that being touched was painful. Due to this sensitivity to touch, I even began to change the clothes I wore. Some materials were now irritating and my new mode of dress became: "If it's not comfortable, I'm not in it." Along with the discarding of my many skirts and dresses went a bit of my feminity. Goddesses don't run about in sweats. *(Unless they're in a NIKE commercial.)* Speaking of jogging, I had begun to gain weight, which added to my sense of unattractiveness. I just didn't feel particularly desirable. When I did feel a tad desirable, I was faced with the knowledge that sex, and the closeness that came with it, was almost unbearable sensation-wise.

When it wasn't unbearable to be touched, I couldn't feel I WAS being touched. It was shocking to me how the body could switch between making even the slightest touch feel like needles to barely any sensation below the waist. I felt cursed. One woman online described the loss of sensation perfectly. She said, "It's like you're permanently wearing a wetsuit. You can feel that someone is touching you, you just can't feel anything particular about it." Besides the loss of sensation being a turn off, the idea of my husband, Mark, on top of a scuba diver, however accurate, was worse. So with it's mental, physical, and emotional trappings, sex slowly became an unpleasant experience, one that I was almost growing afraid of.

At first, my new sex drive suited me just fine. If nuns could do it, so could I! Sexy couples on TV were just propaganda anyhow! Relationships should be more cerebral than physical right? I got very good at comforting my loss of interest in sex with the next best thing, chocolate. However good my plan was, there was another person in my life that was not too thrilled with my sex boycott and was getting tired of chocolate. Mark.

While I understood his gentle hints that things were getting a bit dull in that department, I was nervous that if we did start anything it would be cut short by my lack of sensation or lack of interest. Mark became torn between acting like *"I understand how difficult this is for you, we don't really need to have sex"* and between adopting a red-neck accent and shouting *"Your parts work don't they? What's the problem?!"* I vacillated between responding with a response that is common for most women whether they have MS or not, *"I should just have sex because I love him"* and yelling back *"Yeah my parts work and they're going to work themselves right out the door, you hick!"*

There had to be something I could do. But first I was going to take another nap. I schlepped about in my sweats and Mark spent more time working in his shop. Nearing the end of my first year it became obvious that ignoring it was not the answer to the problem. My relationship was starting to struggle. So, I did the only thing I could do, I researched. And found next to nothing. *(This is almost as good as nothing.)*

Sure now I could tell you everything about men with MS and their sex lives, plus expound the wonders of Viagra, but that did not help ME. The answer of how to get "back in the saddle" so to speak came on Valentine's day when motivated by love and yes a little bit of guilt, I attempted to give Mark a surprise. Since being uncomfortable due to clothing was the last thing I had needed to add on to the pile of problems that arose with sex, most of my skimpy negligees from my PMS (pre-multiple sclerosis) days had been shoved into a box in the closet. Today I pulled that box out and began rifling through the lace, silk, and fishnet. I knew that Mark had missed these interesting get-ups and I had felt guilty each time I glanced at the box. He never voiced a particular complaint about my lack of negligees but I imagined that making love to a flannel bound woman with MS was not the top ranking fantasy in his mind. Today MS was not going to get in the way of a romantic evening.

The long silk green nightgown went on first along with a silken robe that tied at the hip. As planned Mark was pleasantly surprised to find me lounging on our couch surrounded by candlelight when he came home. *(We were lucky that a relative was watching our son that night.)* After he built a fire, we lounged on a soft blanket in front of the fire and ate a dinner I had prepared especially for him. *(Without catching the house on fire.)* Things were progressing perfectly.

However, everything began to go wrong when I lay back on the blanket and felt the wooden floor pressing into my back. At first I tried to ignore it, but the cool touch of the floor began to seep through the cloth and my sensitive skin responded by beginning to throb painfully. Feeling embarrassed and depressed I excused myself and retreated to the bathroom.

Being the wonderful man he is, Mark moved the blanket and him to our bedroom and waited calmly for me to regain my composure. Determined to not let my physical problems ruin the night, I began to rummage once more through the box of negligees that I had transported to the bathroom-in case I needed to change. Suddenly feeling like my old self, I pulled out a fishnet body suit with a wicked grin and began to giggle.

It had been awhile since I had worn the contraption, yet without thinking I sat on the edge of the tub and began to shove my legs into one set of holes and my arms into others. While yanking the itchy material over my skin, I began to notice a problem when the fabric would not stretch up my leg any further. I tugged on it again and then gave up, moving to the other leg. As I did this, one of the sleeves drooped off my right arm. Agitated and confused with one leg in the arm hole, one arm in the neck hole, and black fishnet wrapped all around me I began to see the reason in calling this material "fishnet". I felt like a trapped whale and nothing like a sexy woman.

I shoved it back over my shoulder and then stood up to drag my leg through the other hole. At this moment, the sleeve fell down blocking my view and I began to wobble on my feet. Hoping to get my leg in and my foot down, I thrust my leg through the hole only to find no stocking. My leg shot straight through the hole. Completely off set by the sudden movement, I toppled over to the bathroom rug.

Hearing the loud thud, Mark came dashing in the bathroom to see if I was all right. I looked up at him from my spot on the floor and began to cry in frustration. I just couldn't do this. I had failed again.

"I can't get it on right." I wailed. His lips twitched. As I began to wallow in a full-blown guilt trip, I noticed the choked look on Marks face and paused. It seemed he was turning an odd shade of red. I narrowed my eyes becoming angry. He was laughing at me! A sputtering noise shot from his mouth and he lost control. Mark stood in the bathroom laughing uproariously while clutching the doorframe.

"Oh Hun, I'm so sorry, but you look so…" Mark paused trying to regain his composure. " You look very adorable. You're all wrapped up in netting, like a fish."

Although I was attempting to be angry with him, his mirth began to slip over me and I imagined that I must look a bit like an animal caught in a net, with one leg and arm covered and the other two sticking out. I tried not to smile. He reached out for me and brought me up against his side while he wiped away tears with the other hand. "Come on, I'll show you." He said leading me to the full-length mirror in our bedroom.

I stood in front of the mirror with Mark grinning over my shoulder and looked at the silly picture I made. It was now plain that my arm was in a leg hole and my leg was through the part that was supposed to go around my neck. The strain on the cloth caused me to bend a bit, making me look like a hunchback. Half of my body wasn't covered and I did look a bit like a trapped animal. I began to snicker. Then I giggled and finally blew up in loud laughs. My husband howled alongside me and leaned over to kiss the side of my neck

"Babe, you don't need to dress up for me. I find you sexy just the way you are." He said.

"But you used to love these outfits and sex has been so hard for us since my MS began, I thought you might miss the old times." I replied leaning against him for comfort and balance.

"It was never about the clothes, Hun. It was always about us. Besides, I'd find you sexy in a potato sack!" He grinned with his eyes sparkling and squeezed me around the waist "But the thought was beautiful. What's bothered me the most recently is that you had given up *trying*. Tonight you tried. Thank you."

"Yeah but I look like a netted crab." I responded laughing a bit. Suddenly he whisked me up into his arms and carried me to the bed grinning. (While whisking and carrying me to the bed sounds awfully romantic, he wobbled, I held on for dear life muttering about my weight, and worried he'd throw out his back.) After dropping me on the bed, he smiled and said: "Yes, but you're the catch of my life."

I had never imagined the depth of my love for Mark or his for me until MS entered our lives and turned it up side down. This one night touched me more than any before. I learned it wasn't the wrapping that entranced my husband, but the package. I also now knew that he would be happy as long as I continued to try to find a way to handle my MS inflicted sexual problems instead of just shutting down all together. I vowed to never be that silly again and he made me promise to buy chocolate next year.

While Mark seemed happy that I at least wanted to try, trying was not doing. I returned to my research with double the enthusiasm because, even though my marriage might not end because of my lack of drive, I was beginning to miss sex. Once again the results of my research led me to be frustrated and angry. While women statistically represent over half of the MS population, no one seemed to be addressing their sexual issues. I was led to believe that I might be the only woman in the world who experienced loss of sensation in the vaginal area. Thankfully, I once again referred to what had become my "MS bible", Women Living With Multiple Sclerosis, by Judith Nichols and found I was not alone. Other women felt this way.

Sexual problems in women, like other areas of MS unfortunately, are often not addressed properly by doctors. On one hand some doctors feel they have little they can do beyond medication to help symptoms in MS. On the other some are not even trained to deal with issues such as these. The lack of help from the medical profession and lack of information on the bookshelves can lead many MSers to be shocked and dismayed when their Multiple Sclerosis begins to affect this area of their lives. Sadly enough, as I learned from my Internet buddies, a few marriages had fallen apart due to these problems. Taking all of this information in, I began to compile my own ideas and an article on how to approach MS and sex. In August of 2000 I volunteered the article Not tonight Dear, I Have MS, to the MSXpress, an online newsletter from MS Watch. To my surprise they not only accepted my help but also placed the article in their newsletter, volume 32. Below are a few of the ideas expressed in that article. These tips helped me to regain some of my feminine pride and some of my marital footing.

Be Open

Talk to your partner about your difficulties. In sexual difficulties many people are waylaid by the inability to get over their embarrassment and sometimes anger to talk about it. Some of us have been brought up in families where sex is a completely taboo subject. This unwillingness to discuss sex and our bodies leaves people doing a ton of guesswork and can cause more problems than it's worth. Oftentimes we think that because a person is our mate and they spend almost every waking moment with us, that they can read us. This is not true. You may even find, as I did, that when you broach the subject of sexual difficulties your mate has drawn their own incorrect conclusions! For example Mark had resigned himself to believing that I did not wish to have sex because I found him unattractive! This could not of been further from the truth, but he had begun to develop his own hurts and angers based on this assumption and my unwillingness to be open. Think about it, if you can't open up and discuss it, how are you going to get anywhere? In fact, as I found, sometimes not talking about it can only lead to more problems.

Be Honest

First you have to be willing to talk. The next step is being willing to talk honestly. More often than not when I have been asked to help couples, their main problem was honesty. For years one person had been doing something they really didn't like because they believed it was what their mate wanted. (And God forbid you have a different opinion then your mate.) When things were brought to light it usually turned out it was something the other mate never particularly enjoyed either! Vice versa the spouse thought they always needed to do something that the other person could live without. With both people forgoing their own needs to please the other you often end up with two unhappy non-communicating people.

When it comes to MS and sex even the smallest thing can throw off a good romp. If there are things you already don't particularly enjoy in your sexual relationship then you have already set yourself up for a less-than thrilling lovemaking session. Sometimes just these first two steps can bring about a wonderful change in your sex life. You get to throw old beliefs out the window and start fresh, rediscovering your partner. How bad is that?

So if you're ready to talk about it, be HONEST. For some people this is the hardest part to enhancing their sexual relationship, because honesty can hurt. However, not being honest can drag out or create problems that are sometimes impossible to fix. While a farce is always good for a laugh they aptly point out how little lapses in honesty can cause major problems. In my belief if you can't get past steps one and two, don't bother moving on. Openness and Honesty are two key ingredients to any relationship be it friendly or sexual. If you feel that you cannot be open and honest in your relationship then I would bet it is more likely something else is causing problems besides your MS. While MS can cause a ton of problems in our lives, it is not always the villain.

Explore
Take the time to explore your body. Once you have begun to adjust to being honest with your partner about your feelings, you can begin exploring. Take some time with your partner not with the goal of sexual gratification, but simply to rediscover each other. Start from the head and move down. Let your partner know which areas are too sensitive and need to be left untouched. They will be more than happy to stop guessing! Do the same for your partner and you may learn things you never dreamed. (Like that really sensitive spot behind his knee.)
If things need to move more slowly let your partner know. Sometimes the best thing to do is to keep everything slow in the beginning and then to simply "go with the flow." If you feel you need more or less, you need to be in the driver's seat. You are the only person who knows how YOU feel. Since MS has hit your life you may not know how YOU feel. That is what exploring is all about. Rediscovering our bodies and our sexuality. Don't expect your partner to read your mind. Once again, don't be embarrassed! Swallow that silly pride and you will reap the rewards!

Be Patient
Remember that making your sex life more pleasurable with MS takes PATIENCE! Usually when people think about sex they think of urgency not patience. Nowadays many people expect sexual gratification the way they do entertainment, fast and flashy. But try to take your time. With MS, things are not always going to fall into place perfectly. (Or in 30 seconds or less.)

If you don't feel up to it, do it some other time. This may make you feel guilty, but again, your partner will appreciate waiting for a person who is aroused and interested, rather than someone who seems "half there." If you find yourself not reacting or beginning to feel uncomfortable, stop or start over. Don't rush. Most people with MS have already learned to listen to their bodies when they are at work or at home, but they tend to forget to use this rule in sex. Listen!

Understand

Remember that your mate does not have MS. Sex has always been something that comes naturally in the animal kingdom yet it often seems humans were the first to go and complicate it. That said most people do not have the same sexual problems that MSers face. So while you may be struggling with basic areas of sex, your partner is still naturally rearing to go!

While you may be fixated on your difficulties and roadblocks, they are not experiencing these problems physically. Your mate may be struggling to comprehend all that you are feeling and you may be turning a blind eye to their needs. It is best not to leave your partner in the dark about how you are feeling and it's also good to know how *they* are doing. Try to see the situation from their point of view. Although I don't condone people dropping their own needs to take care of another's, I do believe in compromise. So maybe on one of those days when you are feeling you just might not be able to make it through a sexual encounter, you should try to understand your mate and take the plunge.

Get Turned On

Get your mind involved in the sexual game again. If you're not thinking about it, then most likely you do not want to do it. When I began to have difficulties with sex, I shut off. I not only avoided sex itself but also avoided *anything* that might make me think about sex. I became stuck in a vicious circle. There is a lot more to sex than just physical sensation and if you've closed off your mind from sexual interests your body is quick to follow.

For some people being interested is one of the biggest problems. But often these people have quit trying to be interested! Like in my story earlier I had quit attempting to wear sexy negligees, I avoided watching provocative movies and god forbid that I pick up a steamy romance novel. Yet when it came to resolving my problems with sex, this was a key ingredient. There is more to having sex than just being touched by one's partner. There is also a mindset.

So think about it. Literally. If you find that you have not only quit having sex but thinking about it as well, maybe it's time to rev up your mental engine again. You don't even have to share this part with your partner (although it can lead to some interesting nights.) Be naughty. Grab a steamy book or magazine. Find an erotic movie. Remember, no one is looking and no one is judging but you. Besides, like they told you in sex Ed, it's perfectly natural.

Medication?

Finally, there are medications that may help with some physical MS symptoms that can interfere with sex. These medications are listed in the appendix. Make a list of these if you wish and take it to your next doctor's visit. You may feel too embarrassed to speak with your doctor about it, but weigh the issue in your mind. Would you rather spend a few red-faced moments with your doctor or many nights frustrated and upset? You do not have to give up sex and you DON'T have to let your embarrassment defeat you! Your doctor might not even be aware of the many medications that can help! Remember that you are your best advocate.

Once I started opening up and really talking to Mark, our sex life got its spark back and our intimacy increased! We are willing to listen to each other, take our time, and do everything we can to make sex more pleasurable, so we rarely have a bad experience!

CHAPTER 7

Relapsing-remitting: My Love with the Neurologist.

In the beginning after neurologist No. 1 had told me to see a psychiatrist, I was more than happy to find myself with neurologist No. 2. Where other doctors before him had turned ignored my symptoms (or essentially told me I was crazy) he was willing to find out what was wrong. With unremarkable test results such as a blank CAT scan and EEG, he did not abandon me. But like the true specialist he was, he decided to find the underlying cause. From the beginning, like an experienced detective, judging from the symptoms I displayed, he seemed to know the culprit. Although in the past, it was common to diagnose a person with Multiple Sclerosis after leaving them in a chamber of hot water to see if their symptoms worsened, there were now modern tests that would give a clearer picture of what was going on. Neuro 2 was willing to run these tests, instead of escorting me out of his office with the suggestion of seeing a shrink.

At first it seemed a match made in heaven. He ordered tests including a lumbar puncture, otherwise known as your worst nightmare, and an MRI. He was as angry as I, when the lab messed up the first spinal tap, and he had to order another. When he made the slip before my final diagnosis of asking what I was taking for my multiple sclerosis, I was mortified but accepted it just as one would accept the "eccentricities" of an artist. Office visits were short and he was often abrupt, leaving me to ask the nice secretaries to copy my test results so that I could look them up and read them on my own for better clarification. He often seemed distracted, irritable, and tired. His staff seemed accustomed to this behavior and was very sympathetic. After he had given me my final diagnosis of multiple sclerosis things only seemed to get worse. I felt that since he had caught the culprit, my case was no longer interesting, and he was ready to tackle the next unsolved mystery. Visits became shorter and he spoke less. *(This diminished his already short use of words to the occasional grunt while looking at my chart.)* My knight's shining armor began to rust.

He seemed unfazed by my many complaints and in fact, completely uninterested. Instead of giving him "what for", the term my husband's family liked to use for a good old-fashioned berating, I figured he had some perfectly good neurological reason for not listening. Throughout the Bible many people say the equivalent of "God said WHAT!?" So taking a cue from the Good Book, I kept my mouth shut. After all I figured, like God, he had a plan. I reasoned that he was the neurologist and therefore he knew best. *(I don't recall many people in the Bible asking God WHY he did things. Okay everyone asks WHY and God usually responds like most parents; he puts them in a time-out.)* So not wishing to be put in a neurological time-out and taking the paranoid view, I began to think I was a hypochondriac. Surely, despite the holes in my head, I must be fine, and this was why the neurologist ignored my pleas.

I believe he decided that my first big bang in '99 was my first relapse, so he appropriately diagnosed me relapsing-remitting, then gave me the current medication of the time to slow the progression of my MS, Copaxone. My understanding of the term relapsing-remitting multiple sclerosis meant that after a relapse the person with MS entered a period of remission where there were no symptoms. In my case it seemed I was wrong.

As summer of the first year approached, it became clear that the meaning of the word "remission" in regards to *my* Multiple Sclerosis was not the same as Webster's. Webster defines "remission" as: the act or process of remitting. When you look up "remit" you find: to give or gain relief from. *(So far the only thing I had gained relief from was the spinal tap headache.)* Most MS books, under the same impression as Webster, define remission as a: symptom free period. *Despite the fact that most women would love to have "symptom free periods", the remission in MY relapsing-remitting MS, as I discovered, was not symptom free.*

I felt I had waited long enough for my remission. I watched the months go by and a small nagging feeling began that things should have been over by now. I wanted the remission the books promised me, where all my symptoms went away and I returned to aerobics, carrying my son on my shoulders, and considered working again. I figured my neurologist must be waiting for this remission as well and that was why he wasn't treating my symptoms.

When I asked my new MS friends online I was surprised by their response. I typed in: "Shouldn't I be back to normal now?" and received a flurry of responses which ranged from sympathetic to a sarcastically typed *snort*. I soon discovered that many newly diagnosed MSers end up asking this question. I learned it was a regular phenomenon that a few months after a person had been diagnosed, started their shots, and maybe even read a book on MS, they suddenly found themselves faced with the idea that they may never get "back to normal." Like me, they found themselves too tired to cook dinner, wondering where the spoon was and why they had chosen to caffeinate their cereal. They weren't bouncing back. However, they've been told they should. *(Now for many people with MS, this is true. I just haven't met them because they're quite happy leading a normal life.)*

My contact with other MSers both online and through the local community support group, revealed to me an interesting discrepancy. Most people involved in online or community support groups were never truly "symptom free". In fact it seemed a bad joke that the description of our type of MS even mentioned symptom-free periods. We were aware that there were other people with relapsing-remitting MS who had nice long symptom-free remissions, but they seemed almost mythical. *(Like the MS jogger. We were sure they were out there somewhere but since they were symptom free at the moment, they didn't need a support group.)*

After speaking with these MSers I came to admit that when looking back after my Big Bang in March of 1999, many symptoms, such as slurred speech, numbness, and periods of incontinence, HAD remitted. These old symptoms rarely cropped up, unless I was under too much stress, heat, or fatigue. When they did pop up it became my cue to either listen to my body and cool-it OR... reap the relapse.

On the other hand, somewhere in-between my first cane and my first trip to a urologist for an overactive bladder, I realized that this was a good as it was going to get. No matter how often I rested, lowered my stress level, and took my ABC[1] medication, there were symptoms that were quite comfortable with making a daily appearance. My hands no longer quaked, but the tremors never went away completely. Fatigue was a constant, some days I was tired and others I couldn't get out of bed. I could still walk, yet some days I needed a cane. And some days there was coffee in the cereal.

Remission to me, no longer meant "symptom free periods". Remission had come to mean: <u>anything that isn't a relapse</u>. I felt that I should make bumper stickers that read: *Relapse Happens.* Remission in my world was becoming judged by: *Are your legs working? Then you're in remission.* After resigning myself to using a cane and the idea that high heels would be an attempt at suicide, I was quite ready to accept that my MS would never truly be symptom-free. *(I just wanted to throw a tantrum about it first.)* Like a small child denied a toy, I whined: W*here 's **my** remission? Why can't **I** have a remission?*

Appalled that I might have to continue "living like this" *(as if having an excuse to not wear heels was a bad thing)*, my next question to my buddies online was: How did the MSers deal with the everyday symptoms that were left in their remission? With a response, *about* as surprising as a mime trapped in a glass box, I was informed that this part was left up to the medical profession. In particular, the medical professional in charge of the case. But the daily shots were meant to slow the progression of my disease, not meant to rid me of its symptoms. So I looked to my neurologist for symptom relief. −Insert Homer Simpson saying "doh!"

Thinking my Neuros' reluctance was due to my overwhelming him with complaints about various symptoms, I attempted to back off and focused on my most bother some daily symptom. Fatigue. After checking out a few of my resources on MS, it became obvious that the obscene amounts of coffee I was drinking was not the way to beat fatigue. Whether it was because I didn't look fatigued, or it was summer and he expected me to not be feeling well, the neuro continued to appear uncomfortable prescribing any medication for fatigue relief. My sessions with the neuro at this time were brief consisting mainly of my saying I was tired, he telling me to continue on my ABC shot, and me going home frustrated. As a parent, looking back at my visits with the neurologist, if *my* son came to me *whining* about being tired I would more likely suggest a nap then a pill. I didn't feel like waiting any longer. The way I saw it, was if I hadn't gotten my groove back within 5 months, it wasn't coming back. So I went to my nurse practitioner.

While she sympathetically listened to my woes about daily symptoms, she seemed to feel that her hands were tied. As far as I could guess, if a symptom appeared that it may or may not be linked to my MS, like an overactive bladder, she would treat it. However, in the case of my fatigue, if it seemed a problem directly related to my MS, she felt more comfortable with the neurologist addressing it. After all he was supposed to be heading the team on how to take care of my MS. Wasn't he? This began what felt like a game of medical tennis:

"Well what does Dr. X say? I think you should bring this up with him."

"Well what does your general care doctor say? I think you should bring this up with them. 30 Love, your serve."

After a few rounds, I got tired of being the ball. I was a mother and a wife. I had a toddler who looked to me for support, love, and *lots* of playtime. I was tired of being tired. My nurse practitioner had been with me since before my son was born and helped me through many a rough time since then, I was not about to leave her. But I did begin to ponder finding another neurologist. In the meantime I typed up a lengthy letter to the current neuro explaining my daily battles and wish for help. Figuring he might be too distracted when he was on the job and he might have time after work to read a letter, I gave him one last try.

Unfortunately in the letter I was not able to simply focus on one symptom like I had vowed to do in his office. *(I can't remember exactly why I did this but I must have decided that when he read the letter he would be held captive, so I piled it on.*) I also tried to speak to him not only as a person but also in professional terms. This is another area where I must have gone wrong. One moment I sounded as if I was speaking to my neighbor, the next as if I went to med school with him. *(Most patients don't talk about the "inability to void"; they say, "I can't pee.")* I asked him for medications that I knew nothing about, except that they had been mentioned in other MS books as helpful for fatigue. I never received a response. When I went to my next visit with him the letter was not mentioned. Neither was my fatigue. The visit was once again abrupt and I left feeling like nothing but a hypochondriac. *(Hypochondriacs, like Chicken Little, can be very annoying. Sure the sky might really be falling, but people hate the constant squawking.)* But, instead of continuing under the spell that "doctor knows best", I became angry and depressed.

Not content with the idea that I was a raving hypochondriac or that my neurologist, like God, was awaiting the completion of some great plan; I attempted to discover for myself why he might possibly be against prescribing a medication for fatigue relief. Being the control freak I was I couldn't handle the idea of not knowing.

So I went back to research. According to the MS books, the medicines used to treat fatigue in MS at the time were Symmetrel, an anti-viral prescribed to patients with Parkinsons, and controlled substances, Cylert and Ritalin. [2] Symmetrel, while possibly useful in patients with MS, also had a high incidence of side effects and health complications. Maybe he found this too serious a medication for a newly diagnosed young lady with MS? After reading the side effects, I didn't blame him.

As for Cylert and Ritalin, the controlled substances, it made sense that my neurologist might feel these medications were a bit "too much" for my condition. It seemed he held out more hope than I, that I would once again get back to normal and that possibly if the ABC worked like it should, my progression would slow, and my symptoms might ease. *(Either that or he and the fellow neurologists had a bet going on how long it would take me to drop.)*

Desperate for help, I began to look into alternative therapies. Although fellow MSers suggested diet pills for relief for fatigue, I did not wish to take anything my doctor had not prescribed. But there was something I was not afraid of taking, herbs. So I turned my attention to my herb garden. *No I wasn't growing pot, although I'm sure it would have helped, I had grown various herbs used not only in cooking but also in natural remedies.* My garden, like myself, was beginning to wilt in the summer heat and many plants looked in desperate need of attention. I spent a few months experimenting with these before I finally got a response out of my neurologist. While chamomile and catnip helped for anxeity and muscle aches, there wasn't really anything for fatigue. *(Well except coffee.)* Using aromatherapy with scents listed for battling fatigue helped some but while my mood felt uplifted, the blanket of fatigue did not. While aromtherapy and herbal remedies helped, I did not have the faith in them that I did in prescribed medicine. *(I knew very well if you don't believe you're more than likely not going to get results.)*

Around the end of my first year with multiple sclerosis, the neurologist prescribed Provigil[3] for my fatigue. Unbeknownst to me at the time, this medication was just beginning to be used by neurologists for their fatigued patients with multiple sclerosis. The FDA originally approved Provigil for patients with narcolepsy and its use in MS had just begun. Looking back, this was the most likely the reason that he offered no help fatigue-wise. Because he had no help to offer. At the time when I was pounding him for fatigue medication he had little medications to choose from. Those medications were either controlled substances or had serious side effects. Of course he failed to tell me this because: 1. I never asked and 2. It wasn't his job. Nevertheless, I was not used to this type of "care". Up until that point most doctors I had dealt with were focused on general care. They were not specialists. (Other than my OBGYN and of course he was *thrilled* I was having a baby.) At the time I was utterly confused, and a bit insulted, by my visits with the neurologist.

In the case of neurologists, I have found more often than not, neurologists appear to be more the objective scientist than "touchy-feely" doctor. My case in point was a retired neurologist who my mother knew. When her friend read a medical report regarding a relative of hers to a retired neurologist, and asked his professional opinion, he replied with something to the effect of "There's nothing to do, she doesn't have long to live." My mother's friend was appalled. However, in retrospect, she asked for his professional opinion as a neurologist, not for the comforting advice of a friend.

Viewing my neurologist more along the lines of a scientist helped me understand that although he is a bit abrupt in his office visits, a neurologist is not a psychologist. It is not their job to worry about how a patient *feels*. It **IS** their job to figure out what's going wrong with your **brain**. They are not supposed to spend nights agonizing over your impending depression or whether or not you particularly liked the spinal tap. Another fact I failed to recognize was that neurologists are considered "specialists" not "general practioners." This often makes a large difference in how a doctor treats a patient. In medical school when a doctor goes on to become a specialist, the study is focused on that part of the body, not the patient's psyche. It is not surprising to find that personalities, which are more introvert than extrovert, tend to pick specialties that are less people focused. For example, outgoing people, who love children are more likely pediatricians than podiatrists. (Podiatrists are those people that checkout your feet. You know, the ones with the foot fetish.)

While most patients would be enraged at the lack of "heart" these types of doctors seem to display, they are not cardiologists. They are not concerned with your heart. *(And the cardiologist doesn't care how you felt about the spinal tap either.)* When a person wants to discover and fix disorders of the human brain they become a neurologist not a psychologist. It is their job to know the inner workings of your brain not your mind. It's like the mad love affair between Dr. Frankenstein in his monster. Did he care how the monster felt? Did it matter? No. The doctor was trying to find a way to better the human body not the human psyche. Yet people often respond to this story by painting Dr. Frankstein as an uncaring, even evil, man. *(Okay digging up dead bodies and sewing them together is pretty reprehensible but I digress.)* This argument about how doctors should treat their patients has been ongoing since the beginning of time. I can envision cave dwellers enraged that the medicine man did not pat Og on the back before ripping out his rotten tooth. Think about it. When your mechanic tells you that "Old Bessie's" engine has gone and she needs to be scrapped, he is simply doing his job (not inwardly laughing maniacally at your pain.) Sure you could treat him like a cruel asshole, but that's more likely to get you shoddy work, than a deeper understanding of your bond with Bessie.

Looking back, my neurologist did everything and more for my case. When I needed a diagnosis, he didn't give up but focused on the possible problem, my brain. When there needed to be a test run, he ran it. When he discovered my diagnosis was multiple sclerosis, he prescribed medication to slow it. When I have a problem and need to come in, I get an appointment within 48 hours. And when the anti-fatigue medication Provigil seemed safe to use in people with multiple sclerosis, he gave it to me. Things went wrong when I expected him to treat me with the same care as my nurse practitioner, whose job it is to not only cover my whole body but be concerned with my condition as well. (I can already hear people saying "No. You expected him to treat you like human and he treated you like less than human!" I thought that at first as well. I imagined tar, feathers, and 101 illegal uses for a cane. But come on. He's a NEUROLOGIST. It means study of the brain not study of the human condition.)

Nowadays I do not expect him to keep me for hours on end discussing how my multiple sclerosis makes me *feel*. Just like I don't expect a podiatrist to listen to complaints about how my feet embarrass me or my toenails don't look right in blue polish. What I *do* expect, and get, is his care for the condition of my **brain**.

And for the rest of it, I got myself a great therapist.

Footnotes)

[1] Shots prescribed for slowing the progression of MS: Avonex, Betaseron, and Copaxone are often referred to as the ABC medications.

[2] Stimulants are often considered controlled substances, classes of compounds categorized by United States Drug Enforcement Agency (DEA) as addictive. Cylert is schedule IV and Ritalin is considered schedule II.

Relapsing-Remitting

[3] Provigil is approved by the U.S. Food and Drug Administration to improve wakefulness in patients with EDS associated with narcolepsy. In January of 2000 a study was released by Cephalon, Inc. president and chief executive officer, Frank Baldino, Jr., Ph.D., in which it was reported that 200 mg of Provigil reduced fatigue in patients.

CHAPTER 8

Social Insecurity

Somewhere in between attempting to wrest an anti-fatigue prescription out of my neurologist and the ending of my first year with MS, I applied for Social Security. I had become aware that I now needed some solid health insurance. *(Up until that point my health insurance had been provided by the state and I was never sure when they were going to have a twitch and cancel it due to some new regulation, that I of course would not be informed of until later.)* During my first year with MS, Mark and I were not married, and he was struggling to find health insurance of his own. To my dismay, married or not, no health or life insurance company would touch me. *(Who makes the life insurance decisions anyway? Haven't they read a book about MS? MS isn't fatal! They're not going to have to pay up in a year or even in five, for that matter! I'm more likely to die in a car accident than from my MS.)*

While I wasn't going to die, health insurance companies seemed to believe my "pre-existing condition" was still going to rack up the bills. The way I saw it, if my prescriptions didn't run at about $1000 a month, health insurance companies wouldn't be afraid of me. This was my first lesson in the intricacies of a sticky web made up by health insurance and pharmaceutical companies. I quickly learned that when it comes to people with "pre-existing conditions" health care companies go from care to scared. Each time I received a denial notice I could almost hear the health care executives screaming in fear and running in the other direction to avoid the high-cost of dealing with me. With no-one willing to cover a woman with the pre-existing condition of Multiple Sclerosis and being unable to continue working, I looked into Social Security Disability. While I had begun to master the many changes my diagnosis brought upon my life and body, I was completely unprepared for this pothole in the road of life with MS.

The first thing I learned was that I had not worked long enough in my life to have sufficient money put into Social Security for disability. When I was 16 and worked at a retail store, I was aware that a chunk of my paycheck went to Social Security, but merely thought it had something to do with retirement. Now I learned this money was also used in case of a disability. *(I doubt knowing this would of made much a difference to me back then when I was trying to convince a size 14 she couldn't fit into a size 10 without being rude.)* But it sure made a difference now. My past had come back to haunt me. The years I had spent lounging around with my friends and jumping in and out of college had come back to kick me in the butt. There was not enough money saved in Social Security Disability for me. *(Then again how many people have worked for a long time when they are 23 anyhow?)*

Being unable to qualify for Social Security Disability Income, or SSDI, my other alternative was to apply for what is called SSI, Social Security Income. In other words, the federal dole. I had swallowed my pride before in life to help provide for my family and it seemed I would be required to do it again. Unable to hold down a job, due to the unpredictable nature of my Multiple Sclerosis, I hung my head and began the application process.

The first hurdle was a long application in which I was asked to describe everything from my difficulties maneuvering about my house to my first prom *(okay they didn't really ask that but it felt that detailed.)* Since holding a pen and writing for long periods of time had begun to bother me, filling out the application was hell. Of course people suggested I use a typewriter and type my answers, which only led to horrific visions of me mangling the application in an attempt to line it up properly. Besides, it seemed appropriate that if they were going to ask that I write out my answers, they be forced to decipher my handwriting. *"Is that a k?" "I think it's an "l". I doubt the applicant is saying that paying bills takes "kong time."*

Once my application had been turned in, they began gathering my medical records and contacted my neurologist. They needed my medical records to make a determination as to my eligibility for SSI, or in other words, to help them decide if I was truly "disabled". Although my neurologist seemed reluctant to prescribe any symptom relief at the time, he was more than helpful in explaining my diagnosis and difficulties to them. Explaining the often invisible, yet still debilitating, aspects of my condition to my friends and family had been difficult enough without the aid of medial records. Yet even with the help of my neurologist and records, it soon became clear that convincing Social Security would be near impossible. At my first interview, it seemed obvious that with Social Security, their motto should be: Everyone is guilty until proven innocent. Looking on my cane with an arched eyebrow, the worker seemed unsympathetic and even suspicious. I felt sorry for any "healthy-looking" person who entered the building.

To compound this growing feeling that applicants were treated with mistrust, I was told by my MS friends online that I was sure to be turned down on my first try. But why? The horror stories they shared varied from applicants faced with rulings based on tests results from when they were virtually "symptom-free" to those who had spouses that made too much money to qualify for Social Security's below poverty income levels. (However they could not afford the high price of health care with a "pre-existing" condition and were left to pay medicals bills themselves, often running themselves into bankruptcy. While most people assume they will get health coverage from their work, the number of Americans who have pre-existing conditions or do not qulaify for their work's health coverge yet earn too much to get help from the government, is growing each year. In fact a recent article in TIME magazine adressed this growing problem. Each story seemed to echo the same eery theme, those who worked made too much money to qualify and those who didn't were found "not disabled" after a battery of tests run by Social Security hired doctors. Even people whose own doctors stood behind their disability claim were found to be "well enough to work" by those hired by Social Security and were turned back out to a work force whose health plans don't wish to cover those with MS. Uneasy by these stories, I contacted a lawyer who specialized in Social Security claims, and was blatantly told, "Whether you deserve it or not, expect to be denied the first time. It's almost a rule."

When it came to determining the disability of a person with MS, I could rationalize that the process would be a bit more difficult than deciding the disability of a person who had lost the use of a limb. On one hand MS was an unpredictable disease that could ruin a person's chance at being employable, and on the other, were people with MS who worked full time. *(And jogged no less.)* However while I understood why it might be difficult for Social Security to pinpoint whom could work and who could not, I was shocked by the stories of how they went about it. *(It also didn't help that the lady who interviewed me had long blood-red nails and a penchant for saying "Oh REALLY?' in a way that made me feel as if I had been trying to convince her the sky was purple. I imagined she'd look better wearing a sign that simply said "Yeah Right." It would display her attitude and warn hapless fools like myself who thought it was her job to help.)*

After the book-long application and initial interview which made me feel like I was some sort of criminal for "looking well" and not missing any body parts, Social Security ordered me to attend the infamous medical exams. The first was to be with a neurologist of their choice and the second with a "neuro-psychologist". Had I never spoken with a lawyer or other MSers regarding Social Security, I would of approached these tests as nothing but simple procedures in which to verify my illness. But after all of my conversations with various people who had been through the application process I looked upon these tests not as an attempt to prove me right but to prove me wrong. It did not feel that these doctors were going to "clarify my illness" but attempt to de-bunk not only myself but my doctor as well. *(Of course Social Security doesn't say they're out to prove you wrong, but Perry Mason doesn't actually say he thinks it's the butler either.)*

Needless to say, the day I went to see the "neurologist of their choice", I was horribly nervous. I envisioned some man in an SS uniform shouting, "you have two legz, two armz, you work fine!" *(Funny how SS also stands for Social Security. Go figure.)* I felt sure that no matter what the tests showed, he would pronounce me "fine" because he worked for Social Security and they don't *want* people to be disabled. It costs them money if you're disabled. They *want* you to work. *(Like we have a choice in the matter.)* Once again I became aware of political issues involving taxes, health care, and government that I had previously held no interest in. *(So during the last presidential race I sat shouting at the TV: "Tell me about your views on Social Security, NO not the retired people, the DISABLED people!")*

I came fully prepared to defend myself to this doctor, whomever he was, SS uniform or not. To put it bluntly, I was a wreck. Being stressed and anxious only makes my symptoms worse, and the idea that my healthy looks and ability to walk were most likely going to be used against me brought them out in full force. However since at the interview, I felt that I was being tested to prove whether or not I was a fake, I chose to cling to my husband and not my cane. I felt my cane, paired with my young age and looks, would only damn me in their suspicious eyes. After such a long battle with my own pride over using a cane, the feeling that I should not use it because it would look fake, was unbearable. As if it wasn't humiliating enough to have to ask the government for help, now I was being submitted to what felt like suspicious scrutiny and I had no idea why. Yet.

I found out why as soon as I entered the waiting room. I was not too surprised when I found out that everyone was there for the same reason. They were all being tested for Social Security benefits. What did shock me was my instant reaction as I looked over the others. Without consciously thinking about it, I glanced over the occupants in the waiting room, and decided on the spot who was most likely disabled and who appeared to be a fraud. Not counting the spouses or parents who had come with the patients, there were about 5 of us. From my shallow judgment only 1 other person beside myself seemed to truly have a problem. An elderly woman with a bag full of prescription medicines.

Although I, myself had been subject to bias because of looking healthy, and being mobile, and should have known better than to pass judgment on those of the same appearance, I was still unable to shake the feeling that some people gathered in the office truly *were* frauds. My anger at Social Security's cold manner lessened some as it transferred to those people. How could they do this? Didn't they know that because of people like them trying to cheat the system, they were making it hell on people who were truly disabled? This was a new side to the American Dream I had never viewed before. A dark side filled with loopholes and handouts for those smart enough to find them and low enough to use them. It appeared that some of these people did not truly need help, but were simply attempting to get a "free ride." In the meantime they were knocking the truly needy off the bus.

Suddenly I couldn't blame Social Security for being so damned suspicious. A woman, who had pranced about while outside of the office cracking jokes, had suddenly developed a "bad back" and was leaning heavily on the counter making sure to tell the secretary of her woes. I couldn't help but wince at my own suspicion. Is this how Social Security would look at me? Would they watch my shuffling feet, listen to my slow speech, and think I was a fraud? They obviously had reason to. Somewhere during my fantasizing about launching myself on the woman and twisting her arm until she confessed, I realized the extent of what I was doing. I was thinking like the secretary with blood-red nails. I had decided in the bat of an eye who was a "fake" and who was disabled. By the time the neurologist called me back, I was ready to give him a break. Yet one look at his dour-face had me doubting he was going to give me one.

After an exam in which the Social Security neurologist asked me to do everything but stand on my head, he sat me down to ask a few questions. He started by giving me a group of words to remember and finished by asking questions about my symptoms. He seemed irritated by my slow speech and cut me off many times with the usual doctor's "mm-hmm, now tell me about this" as if he could read my mind and didn't need details. By this time I was exhausted and my head was filled with a fog of floating worries and random distractions. I felt he only required one word answers from me but couldn't stop myself from rambling in an attempt to defend myself from any notions he might have, that I was anything like the dancing lady out front. When he was done with the interview, he asked me to repeat the words he had given me. I sat for a moment trying to clear the fog and recall the words (of course it doesn't help when you have a tall man with a scowl staring expectantly at you.) I rattled off the few that came back and was rather proud of myself. I had the usual nagging feeling that I had forgotten some and looked at him, waiting for him to remind me. But, just as he had throughout the physical exam, he merely raised his eyebrows and scribbled on his clipboard. *(Is there some sort of requirement when applying for a Social Security job that a person must be able to lift their eyebrows like Spock? Do they practice this?)*

After rather ungracefully, putting my shoes back on while the neurologist sat and watched in silence, he stood up and opened the door. As I began to walk out he suddenly asked; "Why do you want Social Security?" Pausing in the hallway where I could see Mark waiting with an expectant look on his face, I looked back at the doctor blankly, not understanding exactly what he wanted. Looking irritated he bluntly added, "Do you want us to pay your bills?" I was stunned. Although one of my MS complications is impairment in cognitive ability, I was mildly aware that throwing a tantrum at this point would get me nowhere. So I tiredly gave him my honest reply "No. I need health insurance. I'm not after money." He actually smiled for the first time and told me I was free to go. I still remember that smile.

I did not leave the office feeling as if I had just been examined but cross-examined. Although I knew I had every right to be applying for Social Security, the way these people spoke, questioned, and wiggled their eyebrows made me feel like confessing every sin since 4th grade. *Okay okay! I stole the rubber band ball!* I had a right to ask for help with my disability, didn't I? Yes. Just as I had the right to not be discriminated against because I didn't "look" disabled. But the part of my visit that made me the most ashamed was not that it clearly felt I was being judged but how I, myself had judged others. I *had* judged the people in the waiting room just as quick as the lady from Social Security had appeared to judge me from my first visit with a cane. As I fell into a fitful sleep that night, I was not sure anymore what was right. Although I felt that I had been treated unsympathetically and even rudely by Social Security, after my own misgivings in the office, it appeared that, having been taken advantage of in the past, Social Security might have the right to be suspicious and strict. Or was I simply being as biased and uncaring as they were being when I passed judgment on the woman?

Attempting to find a scrap of humor somewhere in the mass of suspicion and rules, I likened Social Security's scrutiny to a scene from Month Python's Holy Grail where an old seer stands guarding access to a bridge. He asks three questions of those who wish to pass and those who answer incorrectly are instantly shot off into a deep canyon by a puff of smoke. If you cannot make up your mind, such as the knight who says his favorite color is "red.. no blue" you get shot off as well. The testing thus far seemed pretty straightforward and I was determined to approach my next test just as the knight in the movie. With decisiveness and bravery. (However some knights get easier questions than others and, considering the neurologist's question, I wondered which knight I was.)

Before drifting off to sleep, I resolved that it did not matter who appeared disabled and who did not, it simply mattered that I answer their questions to the best of my ability and get on across the bridge. No amount of paranoia or resentment on my part was going to help move things along. Besides when I thought about it, Social Security wasn't biased. They treated everyone with an equal amount of suspicion and now I honestly couldn't blame them.

Stepping on to the bridge, I faced my final test with the "neuropsychologist." *(Nur-oh-sigh-call-oh-gist. This sounds like the name of some magical force to be reckoned with.)* Since I had never heard of anything more than a regular psychologist, I wondered what this person was. After looking it up I found that a neuropsychologist is a type of psychologist who specializes in studying brain behavior relationships. *(You know whether the right lobe is getting along with the left lobe and whether or not they need counseling.)* Referrals are usually made to diagnose or rule out conditions, and to describe their impact on a person's cognitive functioning. In other words, they needed to see if my brain was as disabled as I said it was. It was comforting that they were at least listening to me when I said I didn't "look" disabled and were delving deeper into my cognitive functioning. But then the usual terror set in that this modern day brain-magician would have his mind made up before I even went in. I envisioned the seer from the movie, guarding the bridge, ready to poof me off, saying "Ah yes, you're Lorna. I've been *told* about you." The neuropsychologist had a line that was even better. No magical staff, no puff of smoke, and no SS uniform, his first line was worse than any I expected. He sat down in his big chair, leaned back a bit, and casually said, "I have MS too." This did not come across to me as a cute coincidence with which to strike up a conversation but as an accusation as if to say "I still work when I have MS so why are you asking for SSI?" When he didn't continue, simply leaned toward his pad and sat with his pen poised, (while I envisioned being launched magically into a canyon), I attempted to hold on to my pleasant smile. Somehow I was able to simply reply, "I'm glad it doesn't interfere with your ability to work." I still wonder if he really had MS or if that was the first part of my psychological exam.

Since I had not been shot out of the office by a magical puff of smoke, I figured I must have passed the first test. We then moved on to what I expected to be more questions about my life and family, like a regular psychologist does. Right? However this magician had more than one surprise in store for me. He began what basically seemed to be an IQ test, which, although I attempted to answer as quickly and accurately as possible, I often failed. I heard myself sounding like a child on the mathematical questions as I asked for a piece of paper to do the computations and was summarily refused. I resorted to using my fingers and staring at the ceiling for answers feeling like a complete idiot, sure that either the chair was beginning to smolder in ready to launch me or it was my brain frying.

Next he moved on to timed puzzles that I had to put to-gether in a certain amount of time. I started; figuring this would be simple compared to the math questions, and jolted in my seat as the buzzer went off signaling that somehow time had run out. At this point, I forgot about convincing anyone about anything and became entirely focused on doing these damn puzzles right. After all I'm a control freak and I just could not believe my mind was *that* gone. Sure I threw out bills and took my cereal black, but I could do a simple puzzle! Couldn't I? These were colored blocks after all and I had mastered them back in pre-school. Why was the time running out so quickly? Why couldn't I move them correctly? I became frustrated at how difficult everything seemed and it appeared my mythical launching into a deep dark canyon was imminent.

Yet as I tired harder and harder, simple math questions, puzzles, and drawings seemed to become foreign. Although In my frustrated haze I was mildly aware that my bumbling was giving the neuro-magician a good look at my cognitive difficulties, I felt very much betrayed by my own body. Abilities I had taken for granted to still be intact, were failing me. *(Actually they were still there but my processing time had slowed. So while it would be possible for me to actually finish the puzzles, I was not capable of doing it quickly. I had become so used to my own little neurological world where taking 30 minutes to pick out shampoo felt fast, that I had not realized how much I had slowed down.)* I thought, if I just had more time, I could figure things out, but my   brain was   busy taking   a   nap.

Our testing time ran out with my slowly plodding through the tests and we scheduled another visit so I could finish. Going home I sat silently in the car, my head feeling fuzzy, my spirit depressed. Was there that much damage? I knew Mark kept telling me that I spent 30 minutes buying shampoo went it felt like five to me, but was it that bad? All thoughts of who was right or who was wrong in judging my disability had left my mind. I now sat thinking: *Okay I know I'm a bit impaired cognitively, but I am not THAT impaired! Am I?*

Although I was now centered more on the betrayal of my neurons than my disability status, I was still curious to hear my results at the end of the next visit. I was not only interested because he was one out of two doctors deciding my fate but also because I wanted to know just how truly handicapped I had become. *(It brings us back to that band-aid analogy. You don't want to know what's under there but you just gotta look.)* In addition, this man had MS and worked full-time. How was he going to judge me? If his remission meant that he had absolutely no symptoms, then did he believe that my remission should be the same? While he seemed the most sympathetic so far -of course you have to pity a young lady who gets beaten by colored blocks-, I was still wary of him. He was there to prove me wrong after all, right?

During the next visit, I was drained. I found myself staring into space while my brain randomly fired out thoughts ranging from "why does the wallpaper looks as if it's moving" to "did I leave the oven on?" While I worried about the oven, he took out a small card on which he began to write. Writing he said, "It's obvious you are very smart lady." I thought "Yeah right if I'm not faced with blocks." He then continued with, "but you've had a bit of a down slide since then." I couldn't decide whether to be offended by my slowness or jump for joy that finally someone, other than my spouse, had noticed a decline in my cognitive ability. I asked him to explain better what this meant. He replied "Well at one time, especially considering what you told me of your grades in high school, you most likely had an above-average IQ. However, there does appear to be some deterioration in your cognitive ability. In other words you are now just as smart as everyone else." To which I mumbled, "Tell that to the money order I threw away." He might have heard me, because he chuckled while he finished writing my new IQ on the back of a business card for me. This little number on the back of his card was my only indication that he had seen some of my handicap during the two tests. In this case I was not supposed to be insulted that my IQ must have dropped since I was in high school, but I found it a bit appalling. *(Especially when I thought of the dumb things I did back then and how brilliant they seemed at the time.)* I absently wondered if considering my IQ drop, I was suddenly allowed to start giving people wedgies again.

I went home to wait.

After a month of grueling silence in which I was left to ponder my experience with Social Security and whether or not due to horror stories I had made them appear worse than they were, I was sent a notice telling me "I had a favorable medical review". I had passed the tests and made it across my imaginary bridge to reach the Grail AND an agency as tough and suspicious as Social Security recognized my disability. However when I went back into the office to finish up the paperwork, the red-nailed lady did not treat me any differently. Unfortunately it became obvious that even if it is decided you are disabled, Social Security still watches you like a hawk, waiting for you to prove yourself unworthy. *(However they can be very nice if you simply want a Social Security card.)*

Thus ended my quests for Social Security help with medical insurance and began what still is, months of lost paperwork, odd demands, and unreturned phone calls. While some people are lucky enough to be left on there own except for yearly reviews, it seems Social Security likes picking on us youngins. *(But that's another story)*

CHAPTER 9

The Birth of an MS MOM

Writing has always been part of my life. To this day my family still teases me about "the Book of the Dead Bird" which I created at about age 9 when my parakeet died. The pages are scrawled upon with my bad handwriting and even worse sense of drawing. The book tells the story of my parakeet and how it's death made me sad. In the end it shows my sister and I dancing. *(Since my older sister was in high school at the time and I believed her to be the epitome of "sexy" I always drew her in what looked like belly dancer outfits with her belly button hanging out. Thus came our nick names for each other "big sexy" and "little sexy".)*

This obsession with putting pen to paper followed me into my early teens where I created a full fictional novel starring many less than desirable heroes in the form of vampires. Most of my family could not understand my morbid fascination with this type of fiction, while my father, who used to design sets for his college theater group, cheered me on. Throughout high school I kept journals, wrote poetry, and wowed my honors English teacher with my willingness to not only do the assignments but also share them. *(It mainly drew moans out of the other students, but I knew not to go so far as to remind her when she had forgotten to assign homework. It was high school after all a lovely time when one fears for their social status every second.)*

In the years leading up to my diagnosis, I had stopped writing. Whether this stagnation of my creativity only helped lead me down the path to my first relapse, I do not know. But I do believe that the mind and body are closely linked and it seemed as if parts of me had begun to go offline even before my physical body showed any symptoms. Why exactly I had quit writing I can't remember. Maybe it was my fascination with the Internet and the many chat channels one could go to, where you can drain out your creativity not on to paper but to complete strangers who will more than willingly suck it up and disappear. Maybe it was being a new mother and focusing my attention and worries into daily battles with diapers, daycare, and tantrums over haircuts. Maybe it was going through a divorce, new roommates, and having a new relationship (with Mark) complete with the usual struggles over who finished off the cheez-whiz and who didn't turn off the TV last night.

As I mentioned earlier in the book my first Big Bang was in March of 1999. Right before this I had enrolled in a college creative writing class in an attempt to get my life back on track again. Battling fatigue and tremors, which up until that point had been passed off as hypoglycemia, I attended the classes and prayed that with the return of my creativity would come the return of feeling "normal". However it seemed a case of too little too late. My body had made it to a point where no burst of creativity no matter how large, was going to jumpstart my errant immune system. In September of 1999, as my first year with the dx of MS began, I had to drop out of my second writing course; unable to predict which days I would be able to attend class and which I wouldn't. *(Besides the professor could tolerate only so many absences and I was averaging one good day every two weeks.)* Once again my outlet went unused as I bumbled about trying to adjust to my new diagnosis and the changes that had come with it.

In March 2000 exactly a year from my Big Bang and 6 months into my first year with my MS dx, I found myself back at the keyboard. During the first 6 months, I mainly researched MS and talked to others online, but as the second 6 began I started writing about it. I placed my first article "MS: the Silent Partner" on a Website called Themestream which paid authors about .05 for each person that read their article. Thinking that I might be able to make a job out of my MS angst and get off the federal dole, I pursued this as relentlessly as possible for someone always on the brink of needing a nap. Unfortunately, publicity of my articles was left to me, and I had little knowledge of how to go about publicizing myself on the web without stepping over an invisible boundary and being accused of spamming. (Sending unsolicited email.) In an attempt to make things easier for friends and family, I began to create a Website that would house links to my articles.

So when I sat down to create my site, the motivation was purely selfish. What changed this were the ideas that began to fly through my head as I set up the individual pages. I had hit a point where I was dissatisfied with simply chatting online and attending local support group meetings, because they were mainly focused on the diagnostic process or those newly diagnosed. But I was halfway through my first year and felt much wiser. *(This is comparable to being 16 and knowing everything.)* I was looking for more specific information regarding women and mothers with MS and began to envision adding links to informative sites on my Website. The problem was that despite my MS bible, Women Living With Multiple Sclerosis, I was not finding a wealth of information on parenting or relationships with Multiple Sclerosis.

This was confusing to me because over half of the MS population is female. Also MS tends to be diagnosed between he ages of 20-40 when women are becoming mothers. I assumed from these statistics, and the numbers of women that I spoke with on various message boards, that it was more than likely there were others out there that wished for more help. When it came time to give my web site a title the name just flowed out, MS MOMS. (Managing Our Multiple Sclerosis.) The idea was to not only provide links to my articles, but also to other sites, and information for women and mothers with MS. With this idea for a group that addressed the issues of women and mothers with MS rolling about in my brain, I decided the next best move would be to contact my local National Multiple Sclerosis Society Chapter. I wished to ask them if I could run a local support group through them. Since they already had a group for the "newly diagnosed", they would love to have a person volunteer to run a group for women and mothers, right? Boy did I have another thing coming.

To my surprise, when the lady returned my phone call, it was not to tell me that I had a great idea and of course they welcomed volunteers to run extra support groups. Instead, I was told that they could not possibly support my idea. I listened in shock as she went on to explain that my idea could be considered "biased" and that the NMSS needed to be open to everyone. "But anyone could come", I tried to explain, "it's just the topics would be centered more on parenting issues and relationships." In response I was gently informed that while I had a good idea, and one that she wished me luck on, the NMSS could not be part of something like this.

When I hung up the phone I was stunned. Biased? Could my idea to help other women like myself be considered biased? I never envisioned it as an attempt to shut other people out, but to open up to others who were getting lost in the shuffle. To me, Multiple Sclerosis was a complicated condition, which affected each person differently. How could approaching MS with the idea that women and mothers face different challenges, than say the average single man, be wrong?

I thought about the male neuropsychologist who still worked full time and *knew* that I had different issues than him. Since I wasn't a man I didn't feel I could speak for his needs, but I felt strongly that there were other women and mothers, whose needs I could address. I was shocked and confused at how the local NMSS could run a support group for "newly diagnosed" but think one for women and mothers was overly biased. I lay awake at night thinking: *How dare they tell me that my idea is biased? Aren't they supposed to be helping us? And where is that coloring book I ordered from them months ago?*

I was hurt. At the time the NMSS was the end-all, be-all for people with MS. Got MS? Join the NMSS and they'll take care of you. I saw them through rose-colored glasses as the big beneficent guardian and guide for those with MS. The thought that one of their representatives would turn my idea and me away felt like having God turn his back. If they, the sole organization for people with Multiple Sclerosis, didn't agree with my idea, then obviously it was destined to flop.

So back in April of 2000, with my idea turned down by the woman from the NMSS, I ranted. I flailed around my backyard, absently trampling spring flowers while I hollered, and even cried, about the rejection. Mark merely sat by and watched with a small grin. My family responded to my irate phone calls with oddly reserved responses. "Of course they are wrong Lorna. Of course you have a good idea." They would say placidly. At the time I didn't understand why they all weren't as pissed off as me, but now I know. They saw the crusade coming.

After all I was Lorna. Daughter of Jean Moorhead, a maverick politician who, spurred by the plight of Candy Lightener, passed tough drunk driving bills. Daughter of George Moorhead, the artistic inventor who could build anything. If you needed a mirror someone could walk through, ask Dad. It was only a matter of time before my blood began to boil and I generated that dead-calm focus of a crusader/inventor.

Growing up "can't" was not a word I heard often. My mother who switched political parties mid-term was not a shining example of "conformity" and my father prided on teaching me to approach fairy tales from the side of the bad guy. While the idea that monsters aren't always bad may of been a bit risky in teaching about strangers, it did teach me one solid value. There is always a *different* way of perceiving things and just because you don't see it like everybody else, doesn't mean you're wrong. (Although your view might be a bit skewed.) For example, the Big Bad Wolf merely ate Red Riding Hood and her grandmother not because he was bad, but because he was starving due to lack of prey driven from the forest by the encroaching village. And besides if she'd been listening to her parents in the first place, Red would of known better than to trust a talking wolf.

So while my mom thrived on beating the impossible my father thrived on creating it. After being turned down by a person from the local chapter of NMSS, it was only a matter of time before I went berserk. If my parents had taught me one thing, it was how to crusade. The best way to set one of my family members off on a mission *(whether they be under one of our many last names Moorhead, McElderry, or Duffy)* was to tell them: "you can't". And I had just been told I couldn't.

MS MOMS now began to change from a site designed to publicize my articles to an organization. If the person from NMSS had decided I couldn't run the group through them, well then I'd just have to do it myself. *But she did say it was good idea-*I remembered, being turned down did not necessarily mean that my idea was wrong or that a place for women and mothers with Multiple Sclerosis was not needed. Because it was. Even if it was only needed by me. I began to buy books on how to create a successful web site and Mark looked into community places where we could hold meetings.

Like a woman possessed, I began to build MS MOMS. There was an advice page called Motherly Advice, with a panel of members from various lifestyles who answered people's questions. Find an MS MOM, where people from various states and countries could link up to other members. I created a message board, chat channel, and bookstore. There were pamphlets, mailings, and phone calls. Mark ended up spending much of his time helping out when I became too tired and I quickly realized I was in for much more than I had bargained for. I quickly came to view the NMSS in a different light.

Their main goal as an organization is fundraising for research, not taking care of the specific needs of minorities with MS. I began to understand the importance of having an organization focused on doing one thing and doing it well. *(Not running off in a bunch of different directions at once, like I was beginning to do.)* The NMSS was formed to find a cure for MS and to provide valuable information to all of us with MS. Honestly; they do a good job of it. I still recommend them to each newly diagnosed member with MS. They have two things they do very well: research for a cure & education.

In contrast my idea for MS MOMS was not to compete with this *(although a few people from NMSS began to see it that way)* but to compliment it, providing information and support for a minority of people with MS. While I didn't turn anyone away, and was always thrilled when MS dads and husbands of women with MS join up, most of MS MOMS articles were geared towards issues regarding women and mothers with MS. *(And I was quickly building a website/organization to do too many things instead of focusing on doing one thing well.)* I had a new respect for how difficult it is to fund and run an organization. Good ideas and good will can only go so far. What the NMSS had become since its creation in, 1946 by Sylvia Lawry was huge and needed. It soon became obvious that if I wanted to accomplish anything I was going to need help. But in the meantime there was a Website to run.

Running a web site alone is not easy. *(Well it is if you were born hardwired for technology like today's kids, but for me, who had cognitive problems as it is, HTML looked more like an abbreviation for Hot Tamale, than Hyper-text Mark-up language. Even that sounded like something Target did when they raised prices, not web-site lingo.)* I'd never wanted to know what "HTML" meant, and I never imagined when I began, that I'd spend the night cursing because a newsletter program froze up. I roamed the house babbling about URL's and hyperlinks while Mark looked at me as if I was a muttering bag lady.

Besides having to learn the language and attempting to understand the legal side of building an organization, I had MS. I soon came to realize why NMSS is not run entirely by people with MS. I'm not very reliable. I may have the best intentions in the world, but that does mean my body is going to give me a break. I may of hit the ground running so to speak but as summer hit and things got bigger, I began to loose step. With the web site I could decide when to work and when to quit. If I needed three days off, I could take it. But as MS MOMS grew to over 100 members and I arranged to begin local meetings (with Mark doing all of the lifting, toting and driving), it was demanding more and more time. Social Security also began demanding more and more answers as to why this was going on and why if I was "working" I wasn't getting paid. *(My explanation was that sitting at the old computer in your pajamas, cursing at the out of date printer, and then taking a nap is not work. It's more like a sadistic hobby.)*

In July of 2000, I grabbed the interest of my local newspaper, The Sacramento Bee. Knowing that a lengthy interview was going to be exhausting I set aside the day before and after to do nothing but count dust bunnies. The idea of meeting a reporter not only excited, but also terrified me. Up until that point, no one outside of the Website had taken MS MOMS seriously. This article was going to come out around the time of my first meeting and I was hoping for some big publicity. Unfortunately, the article came out after the first meeting, which described how I arrived arms loaded with snacks and flowers only to sit with a few of my friends in an empty room. The majority of the article was a dream come true, although a bit controversial, as it pointed out that the San Francisco chapter of NMSS had a group for it's gay members so how could moms and women be biased? It also touched upon my fatigue and the difficulties each day posed for me. Finally someone was really listening and putting some stock into my idea. While people called me and more members flocked to MS MOMS, the local meetings however, remained empty.

As fall approached I was stretched thin between attempting to push the local chapter, manage a website group with what was now reaching 200 members, and filling out the legal paperwork to make MS MOMS a true non-profit organization. Thankfully I now had volunteers, who were more than willing to take some of the burden from my shoulders, but unfortunately it was still left up to me to organize everything. *(I also wasn't about to admit defeat and give my baby up to someone else. I might be wearing pajamas and pleading with my computer as if it had some control of what it chose to crash, but things were not over yet.)*

In the meantime my writing had dwindled to the occasional newsletter and line of code. Despite the nagging feeling that I was headed for a crash if I continued to try to put my limited energy into four different projects all at once, I pushed on, attempting to get advice letters answered, IRS forms filled, and newsletters out on time. *(And I thought the Ssocial Security forms were bad. As far as vague and cryptic goes I think the US would do good to use the writers of IRS forms for code-writing in any wars that should break out in the future. Heck even the IRS people don't always understand what their forms are asking for.)* At what was probably the highest pinnacle so far, in October of that year, with the help of Mark and my MS friend Irene, MS MOMS had a wonderful local Halloween party where at least 4 different families showed up.

Sitting there watching the kids run about on a sugar high, while the moms chatted was almost as moving for me as when I delivered my son. This was something I had given birth to as well. For the first time in my life I felt like a real adult. It took 23 years and a disease to wake me up. (Sometimes I imagined God saying, *"Yep had to slap that stubborn one a few times to get her going."* Except the voice sounds more like a redneck farmer talking about a mule, and that ruins the whole harps and angels thing.) I may of been feeling doubt about the pressures I was putting on myself, but after that wonderful party, I continued to plod on determined that once MS MOMS got nonprofit status and some funding I could hire people to do the work I was trying to do (like mangling web site codes).

In an attempt to make things easier, I changed the newsletter from a mailing to email format so that I could eliminate hours of Mark addressing and stamping envelopes. To fan out the work, I also gave my volunteers jobs (that didn't involved licking stamps), like putting them in charge of different areas of the Website. But even as I began to realize that I was talking to the IRS and it *wasn't* a terrifying nightmare, I started to go downhill. I spent more time in bed and less time online. As I lay back at night my mind raced with "shoulds" *I should be fixing the message board. I should be inserting the advice answers into the web site. I should be mailing every local neurologist office to drum up local members. I should be finishing the IRS forms. And someday, I should write another article.* I had a never ending to-do list and a very limited supply of energy. In fact it felt, as Christmas came around again that the energy I had used to blast MS MOMS off the ground was not regenerating, it was simply gone.

The Website was out of date, the new members were not getting their welcome letters on time, the advice column was behind, the IRS needed more paperwork, and my husband & son were missing me terribly. In the meantime, bigger companies were taking the hint and adjusting their websites to offer what MS MOMS did in the only way large funded companies can: bigger, better, and faster. I hit an all time low and considered quitting.

Quitting is something I've always been good at. At 15 I quit a wonderful boarding school for the arts, at 16 high school, and then a prestigious college for music. Usually it was when the pressure got too high or, in some cases, when I had succeeded and there was nothing left to conquer. Right about now I was beating myself up over the idea that once again I was going to loose it and bail out. When family members began to suggest that maybe I had bitten off more than I could swallow, I forced myself on determined to never "quit" again. I had enough regret in my life already and didn't wish to imagine myself sitting on a porch in my ripe old age saying *"Yeah it could of been something great if I'd only tried harder."* Besides the porch was getting crowded. Already in my mind's eye the porch held Lorna the old actress, Lorna the old opera singer, and Lorna the photographer. It didn't need Lorna the old CEO. But on the other hand my family was suffering and so was my health.

However, like the typical woman who does too much, I couldn't shake the feeling that if I just worked harder and longer, MS MOMS would blossom into what I envisioned and many more mothers like myself would have a place to go. I worked myself into a guilt–ridden mess. I had "shoulds" on all sides of me. (It was about this time I began to fantasize taking up competitive crochet.)

Then one night, while talking to my mother she reminded me of something that was once told to her when she had spent nights fretting over a decision: <u>No decision is a decision.</u> So while I still focused on MS MOMS, I decided I didn't HAVE to decide anything about it, yet. Another thing she pointed out was "Lorna you formed MS MOMS to support women and mothers with MS why don't you get some support from them? Ask them how they feel about you going or staying." She was right. So the next day I wrote a long letter to my members about my feelings and my "shoulds". The women were more than supportive. They assured me they weren't going anywhere and agreed that they were just fine with things being shutdown for a spell. They continued talking on the message board, developing bonds with each other, and I became known as "the woman behind the curtain." This acceptance of what I felt was a "weakness" on my part, was comforting. But as more than one woman jokingly wrote in to me "We had wondered when you were going to crash, you were trying to do too much by your lonesome. Next time ask for help. Now go and relax." *(In fact the members of MS MOMS have always been pretty understanding of my fiascos ranging from months of silence to the inevitable Lorna saying "I wonder what this button does?" and erasing full pages on the Website.)* So I finished the paperwork for the IRS and while I waited for their reply, the web site sat silent, I closed the local meetings, and spent time with my family.

However being guilt-free rarely lasts and my own strong need to work with MS MOMS continued to burn within me, prompting me to once again make that decision as to what I was going to do with it. *(Whether or not it's on simmer, a pot can still boil if left long enough and that is definitely how this felt.)* I sat down and listed what I wanted to do in life. Not just with MS MOMS, but with my writing, my family, and everything in between. During this period of searching, I happened upon the family photo album and found pictures of me as a budding writer at age 10 with my new plastic red and white typewriter. (Of which I was very proud.) In the pictures I am leaned over it in my nightgown with a pencil in one hand, my head in the other. *(For some reason there is a stuffed monkey with its arms wrapped around me, which looks like some bad "monkey on my back" metaphor. I felt very much like that monkey was still on my back, a primate critic wrapped around me, not satisfied until I was at the keyboard tapping away.)* Seeing these pictures only fueled what I already knew. I was not a businesswoman but a writer. I had a knack for writing articles in a way that drew people in and tickled their funny bone. I knew I could be a wonderful voice for those with MS, but first I had to admit I was not a computer technician, bookkeeper, lawyer, fundraiser, or executive. So I made a deal with myself. I would take a year to write a book about MS and then I would devote time to finding the people who could make MS MOMS the organization it should be.

So here is that book. And as for MS MOMS? I failed miserably at keeping my mind off it. The IRS approved its nonprofit status and MS MOMS continues to get new members every day. *(Although I do think they're all a bit nuts for trusting me to keep everything running. But hey, we all have cognitive problems right?)* At least once a week I get an email from a woman thanking me for creating MS MOMS and telling me how it's helped her.

And every morning, over my bowl of de-caffeinated Wheaties, I decide for the 100th time not to quit.

****

RESOURCES

Medications

For slowing the progression of MS:(Also known as the ABC drugs.)
Each of the pharmaceutical companies that produce medication for the slowing of MS progression also offers programs that include books, tapes, pamphlets, and 24-hour telephone access to nurses knowledgeable about the drugs and their use.

Avonex (Interferon Beta-1a) Avonex is an intramuscular shot that is taken weekly. For more information on Avonex, please visit their web site at **www.avonex.com** or call MS ActiveSource (SM) at 1-800-456-2255, Monday through Friday, 8:30am-8pm EST.

Betaseron (Interferon Beta-1b) Betaseron is a subcutaneous (under the skin, like a shot) injection taken every other day. To find out more about Betaseron visit their site at www.betaseron.com or call MS Pathways toll free at 1-800-788-1467·

Copaxone (Glatirmer Acetate) Copaxone is a daily injection, which is subcutaneous like Betaseron. For more information on Copaxone you can visit **www.copaxone.com**

Or call **Shared Solutions**™ toll-free Monday through Friday from 7:00 a.m. to 10:00 p.m. (CT) at 1-800-887-8100

New Additions!

·   Rebif® (interferon beta-1a) Rebif is a subcutaneous injection taken 3 times a week. Although this appears the same medication as Avonex. It is a recombinant of interferon beta-1a and is administered with both different delivery and dosage than Avonex. www.rebif.com or call 1-877-44-REBIF (73243)

Resources

General Medication Information Websites

Here are some websites where you can look up information on any drug which may not have it's own homepage listed in the following pages. Also listed are sites where you may check for interactions between medications or newly reported dangers.

- **Drugs.com** www.drugs.com
- **Drug Info Net** www.druginfonet.com
- **Dr. Koop.com** *(which not only has information but the Drug Checker where you can look up medication interactions)* www.drkoop.com/hcr/index.asp
- **Internet Mental Health** *(Has a surprisingly long list of various medications both for depression and other symptoms.)* www.mentalhealth.com/fr30.html
- **Med Watch** *(The FDA safety information & adverse event reporting program)* www.fda.gov/medwatch
- **RX List** www.rxlist.com
- **Yahoo! Health** *(powered by PDR Net)* http://health.yahoo.com/health/pdr_drugs/a.html

Symptom _____ Relief

In addition to the ABC drugs which slow the progression of MS, there are many medicines to help with the various symptoms a person with MS may experience. Discussing these different medications with your doctor will give you a better idea of how each medicine works and whether or not it is the right one for you. Remember that most medications have side effects and sometimes the side effects can make the medication not worth taking. *(However, many people with MS have told me "If it can help me get on my feet and improve my quality of life, I'll take it!" I definitely understand this sentiment.)*

Below are the medications often used to treat various symptoms. Some pharmaceutical companies have websites for their medications while others do not and the information regarding each medication is best looked up from one of the general sites. When you and your doctor are considering any medication always remember to assess benefit vs. side effects.

Bladder Problem
- Deterol (Tolterodine Tartrate) www.overactivebladder.com
- Ditropan (Oxybutnin) www.ditropanxl.com
- DDAVP (Desmopressin) www.drynights.com
- Hytrin (Terazosin) www.rxabbott.com/hy/hypi.htm
- Pro-Banthine (Propantheline) _
- Urispas (Flavoxate) www.healthsquare.com/rx/urispas.htm

Depression
- Celexa (Citalopram) www.celexa.com
- · Effexor (Venlafaxine Hydrochloride) www.effexorxr.com
- Elavil (Amitriptyline) "· Paxil (Paroxetine) www.panicattack.com
- Prozac (Fluoextine) www.prozac.com
- Tofranil (Imipramine)
- Wellbutrin (Bupropion Hydrochloride) www.wellbutrin-sr.com

Fatigue
- Cylert (Premoline) "· Provigil (Modafinil) www.provigil.com
- · Ritalin (Methylphenidate) www.ritalin.com
- Symmetrel (Amantadine)

Sexual Problems

Treatments that may be helpful in women include:

- Steroid hormones, including estrogens, testosterone,
- Medications that effect serotonin and dopamine, including Buspar (buspirone) www.buspar.com, Wellbutrin (Bupropion) www.wellburtin-sr.com, SSRI anti-depressants, and tricyclic antidepressants.
- Hormone blockers including medroxyprogesterone, spironolactone, and Lupron (leuprolide) www.lupron.com

The following are used for impotence in men:· Cerespan (Papaverine)

Resources

- Muse (Alprostadil) www.alprostadil.net
- Viagra (Slidenafil) www.viagra.com *Studies are being done reviewing the effects of Viagra in women as well.*

Pain"·

Flexeril (Cyclobenzaprine) Robaxin (Methocarbamol) Tegretol (Carbamazepine) www.pharma.us.novartis.com/products/2produ4.shtml

"Spasticity"·
- Ativan (Lorazepam)
- · Baclofen (Baclofen)
- Dantrium (Dantrolene)
- Valium (Diazepam) www.rocheusa.com/products
- Zanaflex (Tizanidine) www.elan.com/products/PainMuscleSpasms/Zanaflex

Tremor"·
- Diamox (Acetazolamide)
- Inderal (Propranolol)"· Mysoline (Primidone) "

Vertigo"·
Antivert (Meclizine) I can attest for this med as I had a nasty spell of Vertigo while writing this book.
- Gravol (Dimenhydrinate) "· Valium (Diazepam) www.rocheusa.com/products

- Zofran (Ondansetron) www.glaxowelcomme.com

These are not the only medications available for these MS symptoms. For an even more extensive list please see the following web page from the National Multiple Sclerosis Society at: http://www.nationalmssociety.org/Medications%20Used%20in%20MS.asp

Remember to always discuss medications and their side effects

thoroughly with your doctor before taking them.

Web   Sites

Thanks to modern technology I was able to find a vast majority of MS information without ever leaving my house! (An agoraphobes dream.) There are tons of sites out there and listing them all would definitely make another book, so I have compiled those that I found extremely helpful and visited more than once in my research. For those of you who are technophobes, some websites have phone numbers listed as well. And if you don't like using the phone, see the book section. (Sites with the © symbol are sites which I have found extremely helpful and highly recommend.)

For Women
ABLED! Active Beautiful Loving Exquisite Disabled: www.abledwomen.org

MS MOMS Managing Our Multiple Sclerosis: www.msmoms.com © (well of course.)

On Parenting
Parenting with Multiple Sclerosis: http://www.msshamilton.org/parents.htm   (905) 527-7874"· Parents with Disabilities: http://trfn.clpgh.org/star/ full of useful links for parents"· Parents with Disabilities Online:http://www.disabledparents.net ♥

MS Help
• MS-EAS Emergency Assistance Services www.ms-eas.org ♥ (Formed by Judith Lynn Nicols and her Flutterbuds from Women Living with Multiple Sclerosis.) 3073 Brookview Drive Cincinnati, OH 45238-2001

MS Clinics and Centers
• American Academy of Neurology http://www.aan.com/ (Has a find neurologist search engine)
• Consortium of Multiple Sclerosis Centers: http://www.mscare.org/ (A very comprehensive site listing over 100 centers throughout the USA) 1-800-253-7884

WEB Information

- International Multiple Sclerosis Foundation Clinics and/or Research Centers http://www.ms-family.org/clinics.shtml (Long list of clinics. Contains many listings in Canada.)

- National Multiple Sclerosis Society Treatment Locations: www.nationalmssociety.org/Treatment%20Locations.asp (these clinical facilities have a formal affiliation with the National Multiple Sclerosis Society)

- Neurology Channel http://www.neurologychannel.com/ (Has a search engine for finding a neurologist near you.) MS in the UK (To place a call out of the U.S. dial: "011 - country code - city code - number". To reach the AT&T International Operator, dial "00". If you are calling to a country with an 809 or 808 country code, do not need to dial 011, but you do need to dial 1.)

- Jooly's Joint: www.mswebpals.org ♥

- Multiple Sclerosis Society of Great Britain & Ireland www.mssociety.org.uk/index.html 0808-800-8000

- Multiple Sclerosis International Foundation: **www.ifmss.org** 3rd Floor Skyline House 200 Union Street London SE1 0LX phone: +44 (0) 20 7620 1911

Organizations

· EraseMS.com: www.erasems.com ♥Monday-Friday 9AM -5PM EST: 617-719-7777" "

· Multiple Sclerosis Association: www.msaa.com 706 Haddonfield Road Cherry Hill, New Jersey 08002 phone: 1-800-532-7667

- National Multiple Sclerosis Society: **www.nmss.org** 733 Third Avenue, New York, NY 10017 phone: 1-800-344-4867" ·

The Multiple Sclerosis Foundation: **www.msfacts.org** 6350 North Andrews Avenue"Fort Lauderdale, Florida 33309-2130 phone: 1-888-MSFOCUS (673-6287)"

·The International Multiple Sclerosis Foundation: **www.msnews.org** 9420 E. Golf Links Rd. #291Tucson, AZ 85720-1340

General MS Sites"

· Ask Noah About MS: ♥ http://www.noah-health.org/english/illness/neuro/muscler.html

· Doctor's guide to Multiple Sclerosis: http://www.pslgroup.com/MS.HTM "this site has many links to other MS web sites

• Living with MS: http://abcnews.drkoop.com/community/spotlight/events/event-ms-990928.asp

• MS Watch:♥ www.mswatch.com

• MS Crossroads: www.mscrossroads.org

Disability Sites

• Enabled Online www.enabledonline.com

• New Mobility ♥ www.newmobility.com

• The Boulevard **Disability Resource Center** www.blvd.com

Government Sites

• Disability Direct www.disability.gov (Provides online access to resources, services, and information available throughout the Federal government.)

• Social Security Administration www.ssa.gov (For disability and social security income for the disabled) 1-800-772-1213

Help with Utilities

Many utility companies have services that not only provide equipment for the disabled but discounts on bills. Unfortunately many people with MS do not learn about this because simply, no one tells them. <u>But there are discounts out there.</u> Here in Sacramento, California we have a utility company called SMUD (Sacramento Municipal Utility District) that offers a "Life Support Discount". Although many people would instantly assume this is strictly for an apparatus such as an oxygen tank this is not true. As SMUD states on their qualifications list: "It also includes air conditioning for all residential rate categories or electric heat for customers on an electric space heat rate, for paraplegic, hemiplegic, or quadriplegic and multiple sclerosis patients." Contact your local utility provider and ask about discounts such as these. (Many of these discounts do require a signature from the patient's doctor.)

In California Pacific Bell offers, among its other services for the disabled, a free cordless phone for people with disabilities like Multiple Sclerosis who can be easily fatigued or have difficulties with the constant up and down to reach the phone in time. These phones come with a nifty hook to latch onto one's belt.

When searching for these discounts on the web I simply typed "utility discounts" into the Yahoo search engine and then looked under "Web Page Results". Discounts on utilities from places ranging from Texas to Massachusetts came up. Another way to find discounts such as these in your state is by simply calling your local utility provider.

BOOKS

- *300 Tips for Making Life with Multiple Sclerosis Easier*, by Shelley Peterman Schwarz, Demos Medical Publishing 1999

- *Enabling Romance: A Guide to Love, Sex, and Relationships for the Disabled (and the People Who Care For Them)* by Ken Kroll and Erica Levy Klein, Woodbine house 1995

- *Living Well with MS, A Guide For Patient, Caregiver, and Family*, by David L. Carroll & Jon Dudley Dorman, M.D., HarperCollins Publishers 1993

- *Living Beyond Multiple Sclerosis, A Woman's Guide* by Judith Lynn Nicols, Hunter House 2000 ♥

- *Multiple Sclerosis: A Guide for Families*, by Rosalind C. Kalb, Ph.D., Demos Medical Publishing 1998 ♥

- *Multiple Sclerosis and Having a Baby: Everything You Need to Know about Conception, Pregnancy, and Parenthood*, by Judy Graham, Inner Traditions Intl. Ltd 1999
- · *Multiple Sclerosis, the Facts You Need*, by Dr. Paul O'Connor, Firefly Books 1999 ©

- *Sick and Tired of Feeling Sick and Tired, Living With Invisible Chronic Illness* by Paul J. Donoghue & Mary Elizabeth Siegel, W.W. Norton & Company 2000

- *The Novel Approach to Sexuality and Disability* by Georgie Maxfield, Northern Nevada Amputee Support Group *(although this book tends to focus on different disabilities and not MS, it is uplifting and deals with ideas about sexuality that most people with a disability face.)*

- **_Waist-High in the World: A Life Among the Nondisabled_** by Nancy Mairs Beacon 1998

- **_Women Living With MS,_** by Judith Lynn Nicols, Hunter House Inc. Publishers 1999 ©

- **_You are Not Your Illness: Seven Principles For Meeting the Challenge_** by Linda Noble Topf, Hal Zina Bennett (Contributor), Bernie S. Siegel, Fireside Books 1995